HOMO AID
T

PETS

A first-aid manual for treating domestic pets, using natural
homoeopathic remedies.

HOMOEOPATHIC FIRST-AID TREATMENT FOR PETS

by

Francis Hunter
M.R.C.V.S.

Thorsons
An Imprint of HarperCollinsPublishers

Thorsons
An Imprint of HarperCollins*Publishers*
77–85 Fulham Palace Road,
Hammersmith, London W6 8JB

This edition first published by Thorsons 1988
10 9 8 7 6 5 4 3

First published in the United Kingdom 1984
as *Before the Vet Calls*

A catalogue record for this book
is available from the British Library

ISBN 0 7225 0825 5

Printed in Great Britain by
HarperCollins Manufacturing, Glasgow

Dedication

To all pets, whatever their size and shape, everywhere.

ACKNOWLEDGEMENTS

I wish to thank the following:

my wife Yvonne, without whose help and enthusiasm this book would never have been written;

my partners and colleagues in the practice, who have been long-suffering and good-humoured throughout, even if not totally convinced;

Dr and Mrs David and Angela Williams for getting me interested in homoeopathy in the first instance;

Sally Hexton, who typed the manuscript and coped heroically with my quite extraordinary and truly awful handwriting.

CONTENTS

INTRODUCTION

I have been a veterinary surgeon for almost thirty years, most of them spent in a country practice dealing with farm animals, horses and many different kinds of household pets. I have been interested in the idea of using homoeopathy for animals for a number of years, but it is only quite recently that I have combined homoeopathy with general veterinary medicine in the practice.

Homoeopathy is a truly fascinating subject and I felt that while I am still in the early stages of learning and knowledge myself I would like to write a simple first-aid book for pets using homoeopathic remedies. In this way I hope to help the ordinary pet owner to make the best use of homoeopathy in treating the early stages of illness in his or her pet and also to have something readily to hand to be able to use in case of accident or emergency while awaiting professional advice.

More than thirty years ago two London business men, Donovan Cox and Hyne Jones, wrote a short but interesting book on homoeopathy called *Before the Doctor Comes* and I would like to think that this book will be considered in the same manner, i.e., 'before the vet is called'. It is not my intention in any way to suggest that this book should be used instead of seeking veterinary advice and treatment. This book is intended simply as an introduction and a guide to the pet owner to the availability and usefulness of homoeopathy as a means of first aid or early treatment, whilst awaiting proper professional service from your local veterinary surgeon.

The veterinary profession can, I think, rightly call itself a caring profession and indeed we are all constantly being told by our clients that the treatment and speed of service and attention available for pets is so much better than that which is available for people. 'If only we could get the same service and attention for ourselves,' is the cry that rings out in so many of our veterinary offices every week. I make no apology, therefore, for stressing so many times that a veterinary surgeon should be consulted for this or that disease or condition.

I have tried to explain in simple terms the various diseases and conditions that can affect your pet and indicate homoeopathic remedies that may be helpful, either on their own for simple ailments, or in conjunction with conventional medicine (known also as allopathy) in the treatment of more serious and complicated cases.

Another reason for writing the book, in addition to explaining first-aid treatment for animals, is to try and encourage you, the reader, to think of homoeopathy not only for your pet but also for your family, particularly babies and young children. Homoeopathy works wonderfully well in young babies and children and possesses the priceless asset that it is harmless. In many instances the remedies work quickly and efficiently but even in the cases where there is little or no response at least you can feel confident that no harm is being done.

Humans and animals have many similarities in their make-up and in the illnesses and diseases from which they suffer. The remedies therefore can apply equally well, according to symptoms presented, to all the members of the household whether human or animal. The same remedy may be safely given, usually in the same dose, whatever the pet may be – a horse, pony, donkey, dog, cat, guinea pig, hamster, gerbil, white mouse or even a tortoise. Homoeopathic remedies may also be used to treat pet birds of any kind and, of course, fish – where the remedy can readily be put into the water.

Historical Note

The history and development of homoeopathy since its discovery by a German physician, Dr Samuel Hahnemann (1755-1843), almost two hundred years ago has been well documented and written about over the years. For this reason I will not dwell for long on the subject but for those interested I would recommend any of the books listed in the 'Further Reading' section towards the end of this book (see p.141). Dr Hahnemann was a physician, a chemist, a first-class linguist and a philosopher. There is little doubt that he was well ahead of his time in both his learning and his teaching, and many of his basic principles hold good today. In his younger days Dr Hahnemann had, among other things, been a translator and it is thought that when he was translating some early Greek writings he first unearthed the idea of homoeopathy. At the time he was very disenchanted with the type of medicine being practised and was convinced that it did more harm than good – in fact, often killing more patients than it cured. He was appalled by the use of leeches and blood-letting that was frequently 'the first line of treatment' for many diseases and conditions in his day. The original concept of Hahnemann's theory of homoeopathy is summed up by his Latin phrase, *similia similibus curantur* (let likes be cured by likes). He attributed this concept to Hippocrates who claimed that he had cured a man suffering from cholera and close to death by treating him with white hellebore, a toxic poison.

Hippocrates has long been regarded as 'the father of medicine' and is thought to have lived between 400 and 500 BC and to have been born on the Greek island of Cos. He was followed in the first century AD by another Greek physician Dioscorides, whose manual *De Materia Medica* contained details of over five hundred medicinal plants. This was considered to be a leading textbook on herbal medicine for over a thousand years up until the Middle Ages. Dioscorides claimed to have cured nightmares with doses of peony which in overdose was known to cause the most terrible nightmares. Hahnemann modified this use of 'like for like' by working with minute doses (millionths of a particle) of a substance that in material amounts caused the disease he wished to cure.

No animal experiments for him; he set about proving his theory on himself and later on his friends and colleagues. First he took doses of an extract of Cinchona bark (quinine) and produced symptoms resembling those of malaria (marsh fever) and then relieved those symptoms and was able to reduce the fever by taking minute doses of the same thing (Cinchona). Hahnemann called this 'proving' his remedy and in the following decades many plants and other substances, a lot of them toxic or poisonous in their natural state, have been 'proved' and used successfully as homoeopathic remedies.

Dr Hahnemann also found, apparently by chance, that diluting the original mixture (the mother tincture, as he called it) in alcohol and water and shaking it at every dilution, a process known as succussion, increased its curative powers but removed any harmful side-effects originally present.

Potency
'The strength of the remedy' can be very confusing because in fact the more the remedy is diluted the 'stronger' it becomes. In other words the less there is of the original substance remaining after each dilution the greater its healing power. The result of this is that at a dilution of more than 12c (one followed by twenty-four noughts) there is none of the original molecule left as judged by the analysing methods we have available to date. Dilution alone, however, does not increase the power of the remedy. It is necessary at every stage of the dilution for the liquid to be succussed. Succussion is the process of shaking the liquid vigorously and this used to be done by hand, but is now carried out mechanically.

Trituration
This is the process whereby a solid substance such as a metal is

ground up with pure lactose powder using a pestle and .
and this produces a colloidal gel which can then be mixea
alcohol and water to form the mother tincture.

Mother Tincture
A mother tincture is the concentrated form of the plant or
substance (e.g. mercury, sulphur, etc.) prepared by extraction
and filtration in a mixture of pure alcohol and pure water.

Dilutions
One drop of the mother tincture is diluted with ninety-nine
drops of alcohol and water to give a potency of 1c (one in a
hundred). One drop of this potency 1c is diluted again with
ninety-nine parts of alcohol and water to give potency 2c (one in
ten thousand) and so on until potencies of 12c, 30c, 200c, 1m,
etc. are produced. At each stage the dilution is thoroughly
shaken or succussed.

All the remedies in the veterinary pack are potency 30c (one
and sixty noughts: 10^{-60}).

Dosage
After every disease and condition that I have described I have
tried to indicate a method and frequency of dosing which I feel
may help in each situation. I must emphasize that this can only
be a guide. Homoeopathic remedies vary much in their action
on individuals and may work well in one case and yet not in
another with apparently similar symptoms.

Aggravation
Occasionally the condition under treatment may appear to
worsen after taking the first dose or two of the remedy. This is a
well-established fact and is known to homoeopaths as an
aggravation. It is not necessarily a bad thing and is certainly not
harmful; in fact, in many instances it means that the remedy has
been prescribed on the right lines, but possibly in the wrong
potency. If an aggravation appears to have taken place, cease

treatment for twenty-four hours and then start again, or if you are at all worried consult a homoepathic veterinary surgeon.

Amelioration
This word means to improve or make better and is used by homoeopaths as an opposite to aggravation.

Frequency of Dosage
1. Urgent, acute attacks – give one tablet every quarter of an hour up to four doses, then one tablet every two hours up to another four doses.

2. Less urgent conditions – give one tablet three or four times daily for two to three days as directed after each disease or condition.

3. Long-standing or chronic conditions – one tablet three times daily for four to seven days and repeat only if instructed to do so.

The exact way in which homoeopathy works is still unknown but it seems to release some 'energy' (called the 'vital force' by Dr Hahnemann) which acts and stimulates the body's own defence mechanisms to counteract the particular disease or condition involved. In such small quantities it could not be the only instrument of 'healing'.

Note: It is worth noting that a homoeopathic veterinary surgeon or doctor using the same remedy that you have selected from your first-aid pack, but in different potency, may be able to achieve good results where your own treatment has only partially worked, or possibly not at all in some instances.

Taking the Remedies
1. Keep the remedy in the container supplied, handle each tablet as little as possible and only with dry hands. The tablets, if left in the open, will absorb moisture from the air,

begin to disintegrate and lose their effect.

2. Store away from bright light and from exposure to strong odours (moth-balls etc.).

3. Each dose should be given at least half an hour before or after food. If the animal will only take the dose with food, put the tablet in a small piece of bread or some other morsel of food which should be as bland as possible.

Dogs and Horses (ponies, donkeys, etc.): The tablets are slightly sweet to the taste and for this reason many animals will chew them or lick them off the clean hand. Alternatively, place them in the mouth, either on or under the tongue or slip them in between the lips at the corner of the mouth and hold it closed for a short while.

Cats: Cats may be more difficult to treat than other animals. If necessary, crush the tablet to a powder in a fold of clean paper with the back of a spoon and tip it into the mouth. If all else fails, mix the powder with a very small quantity of butter and put this in the mouth or, if desperate, place it on the forepaws so that the cat has to lick it off to get clean!

It is thought that the remedy may be absorbed through the mucous membranes (lining) of the mouth before it ever reaches the stomach. Certainly some remedies seem to act very rapidly indeed.

Warning
Remember that these remedies are only intended to be used as first-aid measures or initial treatment whilst awaiting professional help, as in the case of an accident or an injury of some kind. They are not intended to be a substitute for proper veterinary attention, care and treatment.

MEDIES IN THE VETERINARY PACK

1.	Aconite	13.	Hepar sulph
2.	Apis Mel	14.	Hypericum
3.	Arnica	15.	Merc cor
4.	Arsenic	16.	Merc sol
5.	Bryonia	17.	Nux vomica
6.	Cantharis	18.	Pulsatilla
7.	Carbo veg	19.	Rhus tox
8.	Chamomilla	20.	Scutellaria
9.	Cocculus	21.	Silica
10.	Colocynth	22.	Sulphur
11.	Euphrasia	23.	Symphytum
12.	Gelsemium	24.	Urtica

1.

CONDITIONS AND THEIR TREATMENTS

ABSCESSES (Boils)

In both dogs and cats the most likely cause of an abscess developing is a bite from another animal. Dogs are often seen fighting and if the skin is punctured and heals quickly an abscess may follow in a few days. Cats are seldom observed fighting and in fact the awful noises that accompany most cat fights may be the only evidence there is to go on when the cat appears to be off-colour or lame the next day. Cats' teeth, like those of rats and mice, resemble sharp little needles and can inflict deep punctures into the skin and underlying muscles. The small wounds heal quickly but damage may have been done because the teeth carry infection (bacteria) on them which they inject into the tissue at the time of the bite and the abscess develops two to three days later.

Treatment

Apis (Remedy 2): This is useful when there is much swelling and redness around the boil, which has a shiny and angry look about it. One tablet every hour up to four tablets, then one tablet three or four times daily until the abscess bursts or subsides.

Hepar sulph (Remedy 13): This remedy is indicated when boils or abscesses persist or occur frequently in different parts of the body and where every little wound seems to become septic. One tablet three times daily for up to one week.

ACCIDENTS

Unfortunately the most common accident seen in our surgeries in both dogs and cats is the RTA (road traffic accident).

Treatment
In any accident there is always an element of shock and the first remedy to give (even if the patient seems hardly conscious) is aconite.

Aconite (Remedy 1): This is a short-acting remedy and should be repeated every quarter of an hour for four to six doses as a first-aid measure until further advice and treatment has been arranged according to the severity of the accident and extent of the injuries sustained.

Arnica (Remedy 3): It is indicated in every sort of accident to help overcome shock, haemorrhage and bruising. Give one tablet every two hours up to four doses, then one tablet three to four times daily as required.

Rhus tox (Remedy 19): This is indicated in cases of strains, or muscular stiffness after excessive exercise or prolonged exposure to wet and cold. Give one tablet every four hours (four times daily) until relief.

Footnote
The various remedies that may be given in accident cases will be found under each condition that occurs at the time of the incident; for example, bruises, shock, fractures, etc.

ALLERGIES

These can be of many kinds, take various forms and are common today. There are so many sprays (pesticides and weed killers) used in fields and beside footpaths that it is not surprising that animals, who come in much closer contact with them than we do, suffer from allergies quite frequently.

Sudden streaming from the eyes often with reddening of the rims but no other signs of ill health may be an acute allergy to some irritant substance that your pet has come in contact with.

Treatment
(BRITE EYE)   TINCTURE
Euphrasia (Remedy 11): (Euphrasia eye drops locally.) One tablet every one to two hours up to six daily if necessary. See also 3x a day till Better
Eye Conditions for details of administration.
        EXTERNAL   1 DROP TO ½ oz Pure Water

Swellings may suddenly appear in the head region or over other parts of the body as well. These may be due to an allergy and be a form of nettle-rash (urticaria) which can look quite alarming the first time you come across it. You will all have known or heard of people who cannot eat shellfish or strawberries without coming out in a rash or bumps. These are allergies.

If your pet appears perfectly well apart from the swellings, treatment may be tried but if there is vomiting or distress of any sort, professional advice is required.

Urtica (Remedy 24): Allergies may take many other forms in man and animals and homoeopathic remedies can usually be found which are helpful against such things as pollens, grasses and even house dust!

ANAEMIA

This is a condition in which there is a lack of red corpuscles in the blood. The red corpuscles of the blood carry oxygen, which is vital if life is to be sustained, to the various organs and tissues of the body. If for some reason – and there are many – an animal becomes anaemic, this will be manifested by sluggishness, lack of energy and vitality. Paleness of the gums and the membranes around the inner side of the eyelids (the conjunctiva) are the obvious indications of anaemia. One likely cause of anaemia is haemorrhage which may be external and visible or sometimes internal and therefore unseen until it has reached an advanced stage. The commonly used rat bait Warfarin causes internal haemorrhage and if this is suspected veterinary attention should be sought immediately. Homoeopathic remedies can help in the treatment of anaemia and can be used in conjunction with ordinary medicine and blood transfusions etc.

Treatment
Homoeopathic potencies of iron salts *(ferrum citricum, ferrum metallicum)* are indicated in the treatment of simple anaemia. Quinine *(chininum sulphuricum)*, the long-standing treatment for malaria, is said to be useful in the treatment of anaemia in the 30th potency.

Arnica (Remedy 3): Arnica is indicated in all cases of haemorrhage and is therefore indirectly a remedy for anaemia.

ANAL GLANDS

These two glands are situated each side of the back passage and the duct that empties each gland opens into the rectum just inside the anal ring. They can be very troublesome particularly in certain breeds (spaniels, Pekinese and miniature poodles come readily to mind), and may need to be emptied frequently.

The glands resemble those of the skunk and the pungent smell accompanying the discharge can be very distinctive and offensive. The symptoms, often attributed by the owner to worms, of the dog sitting down and then walking along rubbing its bottom on the ground (or the sitting-room carpet!) may well be due to full anal glands. I have heard this particular symptom described variously as skating, tobogganing and even water skiing, any of which words illustrate possible anal gland involvement.

Treatment

Usually it is necessary for the glands to be e.
give relief, but the following remedies may hel

Hepar sulph (Remedy 13): Indicated when the gla.
become infected. One tablet three times daily for up to one
should help to reduce the sepsis.

Silica (Remedy 21): This is useful in chronic cases when a ten-
day course of tablets given one three times daily may help to
reduce the inflammation and irritation.

Arnica (Remedy 3): Is always worth trying in any case of
inflammation when there is pain and discomfort.

APPETITE – LOSS OF

Any animal in good health will usually be ready for its food, just
as we ourselves feel like eating two or three times every day
(some of us more often at the expense of our figures, I am
afraid!). In the case of animals it is the pattern of eating that is
important. We all know of the fussy pet that only picks at its food
and may not eat even once a day but after a couple of days
suddenly eats a good meal. If your pet refuses food but seems to
be itself in every other way – alert, active and interested – there
is nothing to worry about for a day or two, but a sudden change
of eating habits is certainly noteworthy.

The old adage 'a healthy pet is a hungry pet' is for the most
part very true. If appetite loss is accompanied by other signs of
ill health then these should be taken into account and the
appropriate remedy given, or if in any doubt seek professional
help.

Treatment

Arsenic (Remedy 4): If the loss of appetite is due to any sort of
slight digestive upset and your pet literally walks away from his

food as if he cannot bear to look at it, then try arsenic. A few doses of arsenic at hourly intervals can help to restore a healthy appetite.

Nux vomica (Remedy 17): This is the remedy for hangovers and the ill-effect of overeating in human beings and so two or three doses at four-hourly intervals may also help the pet who has lost his appetite.

ARTHRITIS
(See also *Rheumatism*)

Humans frequently suffer from all manner of aches and pains known variously as arthritis, rheumatism, fibrositis, lumbago, strains, sprains, sciatica, tennis elbow, housemaid's knee, frozen shoulder and a host of other things.

True arthritis means that there are changes in the articular surfaces of a joint. These changes are caused by wear and tear in the same way that the moving parts of an engine or a bicycle or even a rubber tyre gradually become worn with continued use and friction.

The two surfaces of a joint move over one another when the joint is extended or flexed and for this reason the outside layers must be glistening and smooth. If the smooth surfaces become damaged for any reason and begin to wear unevenly, part of the smooth surface is removed and an arthritic lesion can develop. Arthritis is more commonly seen in older animals and the joint itself may appear visibly swollen as well as the internal changes taking place that I have described. These changes cause pain and if the limbs are involved there will often be a variable degree of lameness.

Treatment
The successful treatment of arthritis depends very much on the symptoms that are presented and I can therefore only give a few simple remedies here that may be tried.

Apis (Remedy 2): Apis is indicated when there is pain and swelling, especially if the onset is sudden and the underlying skin can be seen to be red (as in a bee sting). One tablet every hour up to four, followed by one three times daily for a few days, can ease the acute condition.

Bryonia (Remedy 5): This is used for the more chronic long-standing form of arthritis which seems to get worse as the animal moves about. One tablet three times daily as required.

Rhus tox (Remedy 19): This is the opposite of Bryonia. It can ease the pain in the type of case which is improved with a little movement. In other words the animal is extremely stiff and in discomfort as it gets up from its bed but it seems to be able to move a little more easily once it has got started. One tablet three or four times daily as required.

Arnica (Remedy 3): This can be helpful in any instance where there is swelling, bruising or pain and can be safely used as a first treatment or an alternative treatment in cases of arthritis to see if it has any beneficial effect. One tablet three times daily for a few days.

Other remedies that may be helpful:

Conium maculatum (Hemlock): This is a very useful remedy especially in the larger breeds who gradually begin to lose the use of their hind legs as they get older. They have difficulty in getting up and their hind legs tend to sway as they move. Give one tablet three times daily for ten days. Repeat monthly if necessary.

Ruta – see list of *Additional Remedies* later in the book.

BAD BREATH (Halitosis)

Bad breath may either be an odour originating in the mouth or coming up from the stomach.

Mouth

The most likely reason for the smell is trouble with the teeth and/or the gums. Domestic pets frequently have bad teeth, or there may be a build-up of tartar on the teeth which eventually causes the gums to recede and infection follows; this in turn rots the teeth. Bad teeth should be extracted and any tartar removed from time to time by your veterinary surgeon.

The television advertisements are constantly urging us to buy lots of toothpaste to clean our teeth regularly to avoid the build-up of plaque. There are not many animals who have their teeth cleaned and so bacteria lodge in the mouth and begin the conditions of inflamed gums (gingivitis) and bad teeth. The scale (or tartar) that we can see builds up on the surface of the teeth rather in the same way that a kettle 'furs up' and this may trap food which begins to smell.

Treatment

Aconite (Remedy 1): This is useful if the gums look inflamed or if there is a gumboil evident. One tablet every two to three hours for a few days.

Merc sol (Remedy 16): This is probably the best remedy in the vet pack for this condition and is indicated when the gums appear red and swollen and have receded in places from the normal line of the teeth and there is also bad breath. Give one tablet every two to four hours for a few days, until the teeth can be attended to professionally.

Stomach

If the teeth are shining and white but the breath smells, the odour is probably coming up from the stomach. This may be due to something that your pet is eating or because it is continually licking various parts of its body. It may be that a digestive upset is causing the problem and this is often accompanied by wind (or flatulence). Heavy infestation of roundworms (see also *Worms*) in the stomach may contribute to a foul-smelling breath.

Treatment

Nux vomica (Remedy 17): One tablet given every four hours will help to settle the digestion and hopefully ease the offensive smell from the breath. One to three doses should be sufficient.

Carbo veg (Remedy 7): This is indicated if the bad breath is accompanied by flatulence and internal rumbling sounds.

Footnote

Persistent bad breath, particularly accompanied by visibly bad teeth or tartar, indicates that a visit to your vet is necessary.

BIRTH – LABOUR – THE BIRTH PROCESS
(Foaling, calving, farrowing, lambing, kidding, whelping, kittening, etc.)

Labour is defined in *Chambers Dictionary* as 'the pangs and efforts of childbirth'. It is, of course, a natural and necessary process, but can be very painful in some instances and homoeopathy can offer some help.

Once pregnancy has been established, or at least suspected, caulophyllum may be given during the last three or four weeks. One tablet of potency twelve or thirty daily will ease the act of parturition or giving birth. Homoeopathy can also be administered while your pet is giving birth and will assist the process.

Treatment

Pulsatilla (Remedy 18): Give a tablet every thirty to forty minutes from the time of the onset of labour until after the last puppy or kitten etc. has been born.

Arnica (Remedy 3): If the labour is a difficult one and there is obvious bleeding, swelling or bruising then a tablet of arnica given every two to four hours for several days if necessary will speedily resolve the condition.

Footnote
My neighbour's daughter had a very protracted first labour and the baby was delivered with forceps leaving her very sore and bruised. I recommended frequent doses of arnica for a few days and the mother and the midwife both confirmed that natural healing took place very rapidly and with a minimum of discomfort!

BITES
(See also *Accidents* and *Wounds*)

Human animals usually fight with their fists or wrestle one another, but our pets do most of their fighting with their teeth. The canine or eye teeth can cause deep puncture wounds which may appear to heal quickly, but beneath the scab there is often infection causing heat, swelling and pain.

Treatment
This can be commenced immediately and the remedy chosen will depend on the symptoms presented.

Aconite (Remedy 1): If the fight has just occurred and there is shock associated with the bites, two or three doses of aconite at intervals of fifteen minutes should be given.

Arnica (Remedy 3): A tablet given every two hours up to four doses, followed by a tablet three to four times daily for a few days may follow the use of aconite, or may be used from the outset if little or no shock is apparent.

Arnica is very helpful whenever there is damage to tissues.

Hypericum (Remedy 14): Bites from dogs, cats and small rodents may be very painful and in these cases Hypericum gives relief. Your pet could be in pain if he is off his food, restless, panting, dull or constantly licking or gnawing at the place where he has been bitten. One tablet every two to four hours or three or four daily until the pain has obviously eased.

BLADDER TROUBLES
(See *Cystitis*)

BLEEDING (Haemorrhage)

The loss of some blood after any sort of accident or incident such as a fight is natural and helps to cleanse the wound but it should not continue for too long. A trickle of blood for five to ten minutes after an injury is acceptable but by the end of this time the blood should begin to clot. Such bleeding will be from small blood-vessels (as we know when we cut ourselves) and is of little consequence. Bleeding from larger vessels is much more serious and professional help should be sought immediately. The blood may be coming from an artery or a vein.

The blood in the arteries contains oxygen and is bright red in colour and tends to pump out as the pulse beats. The blood from veins is on its way back to the heart from the tissues and has given up its oxygen so it is a dark red or wine colour and tends to flow rather than pump from the wound. If major vessels are bleeding, if possible apply pressure or a torniquet while you summon help.

Treatment

Aconite (Remedy 1): May be given immediately if there is any sign of shock associated with the bleeding.

Arnica (Remedy 3): Indicated for nose bleeds, bleeding from the tips of the ears or the end of the tail or any other small wound that cannot easily be bandaged. Give a tablet every hour up to four doses, followed by one three to four times daily.

It may be necessary to continue with arnica for several days when the bleeding stops and starts again, as frequently happens in cases of nose bleeds or bleeding from the end of the tail, which can easily get knocked if it wags a lot.

BROKEN BONES – FRACTURES

If a broken bone is suspected or, indeed, obvious then there must have been an incident of some sort so there is bound to be some degree of shock present – see under *Shock* for useful remedies.

The fracture itself must, of course, be seen by a veterinary surgeon as soon as possible so that the relevant treatment can be started. Fracture healing can be accelerated and the pain eased using homoeopathy.

Treatment

Symphytum (Comfrey) (Remedy 23): One tablet three times daily for ten to fourteen days will help the formation of a bony callous at the fracture site. Anyone who has a broken bone will be able to confirm that the fracture is often accompanied by a pricking type of pain. Symphytum can help to relieve this nagging pain and allow your pet to rest in comfort.

BRONCHITIS
(See also *Pneumonia*)

This is an inflammation and probably also an infection of the hollow tubes that supply air to the lungs (the bronchi). In bronchitis these airways, in addition to becoming inflamed and swollen, may become partially blocked with thick fluid exudates which reduce their size and prevent sufficient air reaching the lungs. This in turn increases the rate of breathing (respiration) and panting and a rasping noise may result. If not checked the condition may well worsen and pneumonia and pleurisy which are more serious can follow.

Treatment

Aconite (Remedy 1): A few doses at fifteen-minute intervals at the onset of the condition can help.

Bryonia (Remedy 5): Any movement see
condition and there is a dry nagging coug
causes the animal discomfort. There is usuall
Give one tablet every few hours and continue ror several days ir
necessary.

Additional Remedies

Phosphorus is a valuable remedy in treating early cases of bronchitis in humans. It may help with animals that have a racking cough which worsens when they go outside into cold air. One tablet two hourly up to six daily if it seems to help.

Kali bich: For the chronic case where there is a good deal of discharge from the nose and mouth. One tablet three times daily for several days.

BRUISES

Animals, just like human beings, become bruised if they have a knock of any sort, but often the bruise is hidden by the hair. The bruise can sometimes be seen on the underside of your pet in the region of the groin, where there is little hair. When the bruise is visible it looks the same reddish-blue colour that we see on ourselves when we get a sharp blow or bang on part of our body. If bruising is suspected although it cannot be seen and if there is pain, swelling or stiffness of the muscles (with possibly some lameness, too) then treatment should relieve the condition quickly.

Treatment

Arnica (Remedy 3): One tablet every hour up to four doses, followed by one three to four times daily for a few days if necessary.

BURNS AND SCALDS

Shock of varying degrees according to the severity of the burn or scald is inevitable, so the shock remedies should be given at once (see *Shock*).

Any burn or scald should be taken seriously and because of the hair it may not immediately be apparent that any damage has been done at all or at least the extent of the injury may not be easy to assess. If there is any doubt in your mind, be sure to consult your veterinary surgeon without delay for advice.

Treatment

Cantharis (Remedy 6): This is a very effective treatment for minor burns and scalds. Give one tablet every hour up to four doses then one tablet every two to four hours during the day for a few days until your pet is obviously no longer distressed, is able to rest comfortably and, most important, not trying to lick the affected area continuously.

Local Treatment

A burn ointment is available from homoeopathic chemists and is stocked in jars or tubes. The ointment contains Hypericum to relieve the pain and Urticaria to ease the irritation and stinging. This ointment is both soothing and healing and should be applied frequently.

Hypericum/Calendula ointment is also soothing and, applied four or five times daily, could be used as an alternative to the burn ointment.

CANKER OF THE EAR

According to Dr Annandale's *Concise English Dictionary* the word canker comes from the Latin word *cancer* and means a kind of cancerous, gangrenous or ulcerous sore or disease, whether in animals or plants. *Chambers Dictionary* gives one definition as eczema of dogs' ears and another as inflammation in horses' feet. Canker in the mind of the general public seems to mean some awful, probably incurable, disease of the ear. In fact most ear conditions can be cured with modern treatments, but even the chronic long-standing cases can often be helped and many resolved with the help of homoeopathy. See *Ear Conditions*.

CAR SICKNESS

This is a common condition, particularly in puppies (and young children) and the signs of impending sickness are all too obvious: restlessness, yawning, panting and excessive dribbling are the ones to watch out for if you want to avoid an unpleasant mess and a clinging smell in your car.

Treatment

Cocculus (Remedy 9): Fortunately we have a remedy in cocculus that is every bit as good as any of the modern treatments for travel sickness and it does not cause the drowsiness seen with so many ordinary medicines. One tablet should be given thirty to forty minutes before the journey. Repeat before every trip, however short or long, until you are certain the habit, which it soon becomes, has stopped.

CATARRH

This is a discharge of fluid from the nose and the remedy depends on the type of discharge. It is more common in cats than dogs and often follows cat flu, when it may become a chronic condition.

Treatment

Euphrasia (Remedy 11): Indicated when there is a continual stream from the nose accompanied by running eyes: one tablet every two hours initially up to four doses, followed by one tablet three or four times daily if the condition persists.

Pulsatilla (Remedy 18): Indicated if the discharge is thick and yellow or green in colour: one tablet every four hours for several days in a long-standing case.

Alternative Remedy

Kali bich: I have found this remedy, given two or three times daily for several days and repeated when required, very helpful in cases of chronic catarrh.

COLDS

True colds such as humans suffer from do not occur in quite the same form in our pets. At different times the many and varied symptoms of the 'cold', such as catarrh, coughing, sneezing, running eyes, sinusitis and sore throat all tend to appear as separate conditions. Treatment with homoeopathy depends upon relating a remedy to the particular symptoms observed. (See under the various symptoms mentioned above.)

COLIC

All of us at some time or other have suffered from acute stomach pains which may make us almost double up. Our animals, too, can have these pains and although I suppose we associate 'colic' mainly with horses, any of our pets may show the symptoms of colic for many different reasons. The spasms of pain may come at intervals which can vary from one or two a minute or be so frequent that they seem to be almost continuous.

The symptoms seen will be restlessness, panting (or sweating), obvious discomfort and particularly looking round at the side and kicking at the stomach region with a hind leg. In extreme cases the animal will throw itself to the ground and writhe about in great distress.

Treatment

Colocynth (Remedy 10): This remedy should be given every quarter of an hour while the symptoms and discomfort persist. It is most important to seek professional advice if the pains of colic persist for more than thirty minutes and particularly if the interval between the spasms is getting shorter not longer, in spite of giving your remedy.

Nux vomica (Remedy 17): Nux Vomica is indicated in the more chronic form of colic where the pain is apparently not nearly so intense. This 'slow' colic is often associated with distension of the abdomen and the production of wind. Give one tablet every two to four hours until relief.

COLLAPSE

The sudden collapse of any pet is always extremely alarming for the owner. It is essential that a veterinary surgeon be consulted immediately. Meanwhile, whatever the reason for the collapse, it is possible to administer homoeopathy.

Treatment

Carbo veg (Remedy 7): A tablet can be crushed between a fold of clean paper and the powder placed inside the lips or under the tongue. This can be repeated every five to fifteen minutes until help is at hand.

CONJUNCTIVITIS
(See *Eye Conditions*)

CONSTIPATION

This condition is not seen so frequently in pet animals as its opposite number diarrhoea, but does occur in older cats and occasionally in dogs, usually after they have chewed up bones.

Treatment

Cats: Elderly cats tend to lie around and sleep a good deal and resist the idea of going outside unless the weather is at least moderately warm and dry. For this reason they become sluggish and so do their bowels, because being fastidious creatures they tend to be well mannered and will not perform indoors unless they are desperate.

Nux vomica (Remedy 17): One tablet four hourly until relief. In addition, give the animal laxatives such as liquid paraffin or sardines in oil regularly. It may be necessary for your vet to give an enema if the condition persists.

Dogs: Dogs that have chewed bones to pulp can produce stools that are like powdered concrete. In extreme cases if the dry hard stool has become too large to pass through the pelvis an abdominal operation may be necessary to alleviate the condition. Moderate constipation can be relieved by homoeopathy.

Nux vomica (Remedy 17): Give four hourly until relief, up to a maximum of about six to eight tablets (two days' treatment).

Carbo veg (Remedy 7): Indicated if there is wind and constipation. One tablet every two to four hours up to eight doses if necessary.

COUGHS

Dogs: Probably the two most common types of cough seen in dogs are the so-called 'Kennel cough' and the 'Heart cough' that occurs in many older dogs.

Kennel Cough

This is a virus infection which is widespread now in our dog population and is so called because it often starts when your dog has been to kennels. A number of dogs in a kennel, rather like children in a school, living in close contact with each other, are likely to pick up any viruses or other conditions (e.g. flea infestation) that other dogs may bring to the kennels with them.

The cough is an irritating, persistent one and although your dog may not appear to be ill and often eats his food, there is undoubtedly some discomfort in the mild case and obvious distress in the more acute forms of the condition. The most marked symptom of kennel cough is that it is little heard while the animal keeps still but as soon as it moves the coughing starts.

Treatment

Bryonia (Remedy 5): One tablet two to four hourly until relief.

Heart Cough

Frequent bouts or spasms of a dry, harsh cough finishing up with a retch as if the dog wished to bring something up, but seldom does, may well be a heart cough. This type of cough is quite common in dogs that are six to seven years old or, of course, older and particularly if they are inclined to be overweight. This cough is not usually as serious as it sounds and may be more troublesome to the owner than to the dog itself.

Homoeopathy can help this sort of cough but, obviously, any heart condition may be serious. If the cough is accompanied by panting, breathlessness or a bluish tinge to the gums and tongue then you should consult a veterinary surgeon.

Treatment

Spongia (Additional remedy): One tablet three times daily for ten days. Repeat as required. There are other homoeopathic remedies for heart conditions, so if spongia does not give relief, then a veterinary surgeon who also uses homoeopathy will be able to help choose an alternative remedy.

Cats: Coughing is seen less often in cats, but may occur when the cat has influenza and is therefore dealt with under this section. Some cats quite frequently suffer bouts or fits of coughing when they crouch down and appear to cough or choke for ten to twenty seconds at a time. This is thought to be due to worm infestation and is dealt with under that heading.

CYSTITIS

Cystitis is an inflammation of the bladder and occurs more commonly in females than males (except in cats). It may be brought on by chilling or very damp conditions and it should be remembered that the smaller breeds of dogs and cats are very much nearer the ground than we are and are often almost touching the ground when they urinate. It is easy for these animals to become chilled when they go out on a cold, frosty, or very wet night having sat by the warm fire or hot radiator all the evening. Such circumstances may well lead to cystitis.

Dogs: Cystitis can occur as a sequel to spaying or neutralizing (ovaro-hysterectomy) and appears to be tied up in some way with a lack of female hormones. The condition can often be controlled by weekly doses of a very small quantity of female hormone.

Cats: Cystitis in male cats may be associated with the eating of the various dried cat foods. In my opinion it is better not to feed dry food as the main part of the diet but to use it rather as treats, giving a teaspoonful at a time once or twice daily in addition to fresh or tinned food. Most cats seem to love the dried food so I would not want to deny them a simple pleasure altogether.

Treatment

Cantharis (Remedy 6): This is the remedy of choice for all kinds of cystitis and can help even in cases when there is blood in the urine.

In cases of acute cystitis, give one tablet every hour up to four or six if necessary, then one four times daily until the condition has resolved.

With chronic cystitis, that tends to recur, give one tablet three or four times daily for four to five days at the first signs of an attack.

Cystitis can be the first indication of kidney problems. If there is blood in the urine which persists and your pet is off-colour or suddenly drinking large quantities of water, then you should see your veterinary surgeon as soon as possible.

DANDRUFF (SCURF)
(See also *Skin Conditions*)

The production of large or small scales which peel away from the surface of the skin sometimes in large quantities. The sudden appearance of a good deal of dandruff or scurf may well indicate an underlying or more deep-seated problem which will need investigation if it continues.

Treatment

Arsenic (Remedy 4): Give one tablet three times daily for up to one week and then cease treatment for one to two weeks to see if there is any improvement. Any skin condition is likely to take some days or even weeks to respond to treatment, so please be patient.

DERMATITIS
(See also *Skin Conditions*)

This is an inflammation of the surface layers of the skin which causes irritation. The irritation in turn leads to scratching or rubbing of the affected area which may then become infected. Alternatively, the animal may lick the affected area continually, making it red and sore and producing eczema. (See *Skin Conditions*.)

DIARRHOEA

The word diarrhoea is very familiar to us all and we have all suffered from this condition at some time or other. Diarrhoea means the passing of liquid motions (faeces or stools). In treating diarrhoea homoeopathically, it is often advantageous to try and ascertain the cause or reason for the condition arising. (See *Enteritis* for treatment.)

DISTEMPER/HARDPAD

This is possibly the disease of dogs (also ferrets and mink) that is best known to the general public, probably because there is no comparable condition in human beings. Distemper is a virus disease and the virus itself is quite closely associated with the virus that causes measles.

Distemper used to be the scourge of the dog population and still occurs where dogs congregate together, as in stray dogs' homes and large boarding kennels, unless they are already protected by vaccination. Fortunately excellent vaccines are available today and there is no reason why any dog should have to suffer this terrible disease. In fact, anybody who has seen distemper in the dog or tried to nurse a case would never want to see another dog have to go through the various stages of this condition. This disease usually terminates in death or at the least some permanent nerve damage causing involuntary twitchings of part of the body.

The symptoms are many and various and veterinary treatment is essential if there is to be any hope of the dog surviving an attack. Homoeopathy can only help with the individual symptoms, some of which I have listed here, and the appropriate remedy will be found under the relevant section of this book (e.g. *Running Eyes, Cough*, etc.).

Symptoms of Distemper

1. The temperature fluctuates up and down during the course of the disease which may take up to three months before limited recovery or death takes place (see *Fever*).

2. Running eyes: the discharge may be watery in the first instance but later becomes thick, yellow and purulent (see *Eye Conditions* – conjunctivitis).

3. Running nose: this discharge, too, becomes thick and purulent and can form crusts over the nostrils which may block them completely. The crusts should be removed gently with warm water to which a little Hypercal lotion may be added (see *Catarrh*).

4. Cough: this symptom is seen in the hardpad form of distemper. Incidentally, the name hardpad is rather confusing because the hardening of the pads, which eventually peel off if the animal survives, is one of the last symptoms to appear (see *Coughs*).

5. Tonsillitis: inflammation of the tonsils and the other glands at the back of the mouth causes difficulty in swallowing and possibly also salivation (dribbling) (see *Tonsillitis*).

6. Loss of appetite: this is one of the first signs of ill health in almost all diseases of our domestic animals, but nevertheless is one to take into account (see *Appetite – Loss of*).

7. Diarrhoea: another symptom seen as the disease progresses and more often in the hardpad form of distemper (see *Enteritis*).

8. Pneumonia: pneumonia develops five to six weeks from the onset of the disease and after a period when the dog has often seemed a little better and even started to eat again fairly well. In my experience if the dog develops pneumonia then the chances of survival and recovery are only slight (see *Pneumonia*).

9. Nervous symptoms: nervous symptoms, as with the hardening of the pads, appear late in the course of the disease. These symptoms may take the form of fits, or chorea, an involuntary form of twitching of one of the limbs which may be permanent, or paralysis of the hind limbs – paraplegia. Conium maculatum (hemlock), given two or three times daily for up to a week at a time can help to relieve the symptom of paraplegia. (See *Fits* and *Nervous Conditions*).

Footnote
Homoeopathic vaccines for distemper, hepatitis and leptospirosis are available and I understand that they are effective but I have no experience of their use.

DYSENTERY
(See *Enteritis*)

Diarrhoea containing blood.

EAR CONDITIONS

Ear problems of various kinds bring many pets to our surgeries in the course of a week.

Ear conditions require topical applications of various types which may be allopathic (ordinary medicines) or homoeopathic. The many allopathic preparations available can be used locally quite safely in conjunction with homoeopathic remedies given by mouth at the same time.

Inflammation – Otitis
A reddening and irritation of the ear canal but with little sign of wax or discharge of any sort.

Treatment

Apis mel (Remedy 2): Apis is useful if the folds in the canal are swollen and inclined to rub against one another. One tablet every two hours up to four, then one tablet three times daily for a few days until relief.

Topical application

Hypercal lotion: Several drops two or three times daily for a few days.

Infected Otitis
Animals naturally scratch and rub their ears if they become sore and in this way may introduce dirt and set up infection. In such cases there is often a sticky, dirty-looking discharge possibly accompanied by an offensive smell.

Treatment

Hepar sulph (Remedy 13): Give a tablet every two hours up to four doses, then one three times daily for three to four days.

Alternative Remedy

Graphites: Dose as for Hepar sulph. Useful when there is a lot of smelly discharge.

Pain in the Ear

The slightest touch or even just brushing past the ear causes the animal to yelp or make a noise and move away sharply. Sometimes it will cry out suddenly when it is scratching its ear.

Treatment

Chamomilla (Remedy 8): Give a tablet every half to one hour in cases of extreme discomfort or three to four times daily until relief.

Parasitic Otitis

Parasitic otitis can occur in dogs, cats and quite commonly in rabbits. In this condition tiny mites living in the wax are present in the ear and their activity promotes excess wax production. This wax is dark brown in colour and may smell unpleasant. The mites naturally irritate the animal's ear and cause prolonged, vigorous scratching, shaking of the head and sometimes the head is held hanging down to the affected side. The mites are just visible to the naked eye as white moving dots, but can readily be seen with a hand lens or auriscope.

Treatment

It is, of course, necessary in the first place to kill the mites that are living in the wax. Your veterinary surgeon may apply a wax solvent to soften the wax and will then supply suitable ear drops to kill the mites.

The various homoeopathic remedies outlined above may be used in addition to the ear drops, the exact remedy being selected according to the main symptoms presented (e.g. infected – Hepar sulph; painful – Chamomilla).

Eczema of the Ear

Eczema will be described more fully under the heading *Skin Conditions*. If the ear flap and the top of the canal are very red, inflamed and have a wet, sore appearance, this is probably acute eczema.

Treatment

Merc sol (Remedy 16): One tablet two hourly during the first day, followed by one four hourly for a few days.

Middle Ear Disease

This happens when the membrane at the base of the external canal becomes damaged and an infection enters the middle part of the ear. The middle ear is very much concerned with the process of hearing and is a delicate structure. It has a connecting tube with the back of the mouth and if this becomes blocked with catarrh, as sometimes happens with a heavy cold, temporary deafness may result.

Treatment

Hepar sulph (Remedy 13): For offensive-smelling discharges from the ear. One tablet two hourly up to four, then one three times daily.

Merc cor (Remedy 15): This remedy is useful in the treatment of chronic infection of the middle ear. One tablet every two hours up to four tablets, then one three times daily for seven to ten days if necessary.

Aural Haematoma

This is a 'blood blister' which forms in the flap of the ear. It usually occurs because there is some trouble inside the ear itself causing the animal to scratch or shake its head vigorously, thus damaging small blood vessels in the ear flap. The swelling can occupy the whole of the ear flap and may need surgery to correct it.

Treatment
For the small haematoma, to try to prevent further haemorrhage, and for the elderly dog which may not be a good risk for an operation.

Arnica (Remedy 3): One tablet three times daily for seven to fourteen days or longer, until the swelling becomes reduced.

ECZEMA OF THE SKIN
(See *Skin Conditions*)

ENTERITIS

Enteritis means the inflammation of the intestines or bowels. The effect of such an inflammation is to speed up the progress of the food through the bowel so that liquid stools (diarrhoea) result. There are many reasons why diarrhoea develops and it is important to try and find out if it is caused by something eaten in the usual diet, or something scavenged, or from an infection of some kind.

Dogs: Acute Diarrhoea
Dogs on the whole are not fussy feeders and those (especially puppies) who tend to eat anything and everything are quite likely to have their insides upset, resulting in an attack of diarrhoea. The diarrhoea may or may not be accompanied by vomiting.

Treatment

Arsenic (Remedy 4): This remedy is indicated when vomiting and diarrhoea occur at the same time, usually with very little warning. The vomiting can be very frequent and there is usually a great desire for water which is vomited back almost immediately. The diarrhoea is usually accompanied by extreme restlessness and the animal feels cold to the touch. One tablet every quarter of an hour up to eight doses if necessary until the vomiting ceases, and then one three or four times daily for two to three days should also stop the diarrhoea.

Merc cor (Remedy 15): When there is frequent diarrhoea with a lot of straining but no vomiting, this remedy is often helpful. One tablet two hourly up to four doses, then one three times daily for two to three days should be sufficient.

Chronic Diarrhoea
This is a fairly common condition in quite a few breeds of dogs and the diarrhoea tends to recur frequently for no apparent reason. It will usually clear up with the use of ordinary medicines but returns soon after the treatment is completed. Samples taken in such cases usually reveal little or no infection present and the reasons for these persistent attacks of diarrhoea remain obscure.

Treatment
In such cases it is often necessary to try one or two remedies in order to find the correct one.

Merc cor (Remedy 15); *Merc sol* (Remedy 16); *Sulphur* (Remedy 22): One tablet three times daily for up to a week may be tried initially to see what response, if any, can be achieved.

Alternative Remedy
I have found the use of Croton tiglium (croton oil seeds) helpful in the treatment of a number of chronic diarrhoea cases when there is a lot of watery motion frequently passed. One tablet three times daily for up to a week may well help to resolve this tiresome condition. The treatment may have to be repeated until the condition is brought under control.

Haemorrhagic Enteritis (Dysentery)
In such cases the inflammation of the bowel is so severe that

some of the bowel lining has been 'burned' away and bleeding occurs. This blood colours the diarrhoea and has a characteristic pungent odour. This condition can be very serious indeed.

If the bloodstained stool is accompanied by vomiting, which may also be bloodstained, then veterinary help must be sought immediately, particularly if your pet feels cold and clammy to the touch and is in a state of semi- or complete collapse. Persistent enteritis and diarrhoea causes rapid dehydration of the animal and it is necessary for the body fluids and essential salts to be replaced by injections or drips to restore what is known as the electrolyte balance. If this is not done then the patient will die.

Treatment
(of the not so severe case, when the animal is passing some blood but is not off-colour, off his food or dull and lying about)

Merc Cor (Remedy 15): One tablet every quarter of an hour until the condition improves, followed by one three times daily for several days until health is restored.

Canine Parvovirus
Canine Parvovirus is a new virus disease of dogs that first appeared in many different parts of the world in 1978. In young puppies under five weeks old it affects the heart muscle, causing heart failure, weakness, sudden collapse and death. In older puppies and adult dogs it causes severe vomiting and diarrhoea with often very rapid dehydration.

Treatment
Mercurius corrosivus or arsenic may be tried in conjunction with fluid therapy, but many cases, unfortunately, do not respond to treatment.

Vaccination
Ordinary vaccinations against Parvovirus are now freely available and very effective. It is also possible to use a homoeopathic oral

vaccine if this is preferred, but I have no experience of this preparation.

Cats: Acute Diarrhoea

The best-known disease causing diarrhoea in cats is feline enteritis (feline panleucopenia) which is due to a parvovirus related to the one described previously that has attacked dogs in recent years.

It is mainly a disease of young cats characterized by profuse watery diarrhoea, vomiting, loss of appetite and dullness which can soon lead to extreme depression, collapse and death. Treatment by your veterinary surgeon must be given as soon as the first signs of ill health are spotted.

Vaccines against infectious feline enteritis have been available for some years and are very effective. A homoeopathic oral vaccine may be used if preferred to the ordinary vaccines, but I have no experience of this.

Homoeopathic Treatment

Arsenic (Remedy 4): For simultaneous vomiting and diarrhoea give one tablet every quarter of an hour up to eight doses if required, then one three to four times daily until the symptoms stop.

Merc cor (Remedy 15); *Merc sol* (Remedy 16): For acute diarrhoea cases when the cat does not appear to be ill apart from the very loose stools. There is often thirst associated with this type of diarrhoea and a cat which may not normally drink water will be found at the water bowl or in the sink etc. Give one tablet two hourly up to four doses, then one tablet two or three times daily until a normal motion is produced.

Chronic Diarrhoea

Some cats suffer from a chronic form of diarrhoea and permanently pass unformed stools. In many cases this condition may not be observed by the owner for months because cats tend to be clean animals and will only pass a motion indoors if they cannot get out for some reason.

Treatment
In such cases it will be necessary to find a remedy that resolves the condition in your cat. Any of the following remedies may be tried:

Arsenic (Remedy 4); *Merc Cor* (Remedy 15); *Merc Sol* (Remedy 16); *Sulphur* (Remedy 22): One tablet should be given two or three times daily for up to a week to see if any response can be achieved.

EYE CONDITIONS

The eyes are just as important to an animal as ours are to us. The eye is a very delicate structure and for this reason I must stress that any eye condition may be potentially serious and should therefore be investigated by your veterinary surgeon. Immediate treatment can often prevent permanent damage to the eye or even blindness.

Homoeopathy can be used at the same time as conventional medicines in the more acute conditions. In addition it has a lot to offer in the more long-standing and less serious conditions.

Conjunctivitis
Inflammation of the conjunctiva which is the membrane lining the inner side of the eyelids and the external surface of the eyeball (the cornea).

Acute Conjunctivitis
The inflammation is often accompanied by a discharge which may be clear or become thick and yellow/white in colour.

Topical application
For the clear discharge I have found euphrasia eye drops very

effective. The concentrated drops can be purchased from a homoeopathic chemist and one drop in an eye-bath or eggcup full of warm (previously boiled) water is all that is required. Dip a piece of clean cotton-wool in the solution and squeeze it out over the eye so that drops bathe the eyeball. Repeat one to three times daily as necessary.

Treatment

Treatment by mouth may be given in addition to the use of euphrasia eye drops or proprietary eye ointments.

Apis Mel (Remedy 2): In the sudden, acute attack when there is swelling of the eyelids. One tablet two hourly up to four or five doses, then one three times daily for two to three days.

Arsenic (Remedy 4): This remedy may be considered where the tears are scalding the skin beneath the eye (a condition seen in poodles and sometimes in other breeds). One tablet every four hours (three or four daily) for a few days.

Euphrasia (Remedy 11): Useful when there is profuse production of tears and marked reddening of the inner side of the lids. One tablet every two hours up to four doses, followed by one tablet three or four times daily until relief.

Sulphur (Remedy 22): In some cases there is reddening of the lids but not much production of tears or any real signs of infection. One tablet three times daily for two to three days.

Chronic Conjunctivitis

This condition is not usually serious but tends to persist or recur as soon as any form of treatment is completed.

Euphrasia (Remedy 11): One tablet three or four times daily for up to a week and repeated when necessary if it seems to relieve the condition. Euphrasia eye drops made up as indicated for acute conjunctivitis can be helpful and may be used as little or as often as required.

Silica (Remedy 21): One tablet three times daily for up to a week in cases where conjunctivitis persists after an injury to the eye or from a foreign body irritating the surface of the eye.

Cataract

An opacity of the lens of the eye. Cataract is seen more often as animals get older and occurs more in dogs than cats. The change in the lens is irreversible but the process may be very slow, and the animal will have time to adapt to the new situation of approaching blindness as it develops.

Treatment
This can only be of a palliative or temporary nature.

Euphrasia (Remedy 11): One tablet three times daily for ten to fourteen days if there is tear formation as the condition develops.

Silica (Remedy 21): This may be helpful in delaying the progress of a cataract but it would have to be taken for weeks or months. One tablet once or twice daily.

Corneal Ulcer

The eyes of many animals have extra protection in the form of a third eyelid which lies in the inner corner of the eye (nearest to the nose). This third eyelid can sometimes protrude and almost cover the eye, particularly in cats if they are below par or lose weight very quickly. This eyelid helps to prevent injury to the cornea or front surface of the eye. In spite of this safeguard the eye may become damaged by a scratch or other injury which makes a crater on the eye surface. This injury causes irritation and the animal tries to scratch it and soon introduces infection. Such an injury is known as a corneal ulcer.

In order to repair such damage, blood-vessels have to grow out from the edge of the eyeball, remain there while the healing process takes place and then recede. The whole process may take several weeks.

Treatment

Symphytum (Remedy 23): For any painful blow on the eyeball causing bruising or damage to the cornea. One tablet every two hours up to four, then one three or four times daily.

Arnica (Remedy 3): For bruising of the eye this remedy, too, can be useful. One tablet three times daily for a few days as soon as the injury occurs.

Silica (Remedy 21): One tablet twice daily for ten to fourteen days.

Topical Application
Diluted tincture of symphytum (one drop in an eye-bath of boiled warm water) may be used to bathe the eye as an alternative to euphrasia in this condition.

Footnote
Homoeopathy, as we have said, is treating like with like and here we have a simple example to demonstrate this principle. When allium cepa, the ordinary onion, is being peeled it is able to force tears from the eyes; therefore a homoeopathic potency of onion can be useful in treating some cases of persistent tear production, known as lachrymation.

FALSE OR PHANTOM PREGNANCY

False pregnancy is a curious condition seen in some bitches eight to nine weeks after their season and the symptoms can be various and tiresome for both dog and owner.

Mammary gland development and milk production are two of the common signs of false pregnancy. These may be accompanied by whining, digging, restlessness and the desire to 'make a bed' and the taking of socks or other small household articles to the bed. These are then guarded or 'nursed' and sometimes the normally quiet bitch can become quite aggressive and growls as she protects her imaginary young.

Treatment

Pulsatilla (Remedy 18): One tablet three times daily for seven to ten days should help to correct this condition.

FEAR, FRIGHT, APPREHENSION, PANIC

There are many reasons why your pet may be frightened and it is important to find the cause if you can and remove it if possible. Loud noises such as fireworks, cars backfiring or guns going off certainly frighten a lot of our household pets.

Treatment

Aconite (Remedy 1): Fear following any sort of shock or accident. One tablet every quarter of an hour until calmness is restored (up to four or six doses).

Arsenicum album (Remedy 4): For the fright which has occurred when the animal has been left on its own, particularly if it has passed a motion out of fear. One tablet every fifteen minutes up to four doses, then one four hourly if necessary.

Gelsemium (Remedy 12): When the animal is literally 'shaking with fright' and may have wet the floor and made a 'mess'. One tablet every hour up to four doses.

Pulsatilla (Remedy 18): Pulsatilla can be given to the dog that dislikes being left in the house on its own. Some of these dogs bark all the time that their owner is out and may well upset the neighbours. One tablet given twice daily the day before and on the day that you will be away can help to prevent this situation.

Scutellaria (Remedy 20): This remedy is useful when your pet's nature suddenly seems to change, possibly after moving house, or a change of routine which necessitates leaving the animal alone all day. A quiet animal becomes noisy, destructive, and very restless and unable to settle down. Give one tablet twice daily for two to three days, then cease treatment to see if calmness is restored. Repeat if necessary after a week.

Alternative Remedy

Borax: This is particularly effective when loud noises such as those heard on Bonfire Night are expected. If possible, give a tablet three times daily for several days before the calming action is required.

FEVER

When the temperature is raised above normal it usually indicates that the activity of the body's defence mechanisms has increased for some reason, probably because of an infection of some kind. The raised temperature therefore is not in itself a bad thing and in fact the temperature that falls rapidly and finishes up well below normal is often much more serious.

Fever is usually accompanied by loss of appetite, dullness, shivering and moving about in a sluggish manner. Increased rate of breathing or panting soon follow and there is often great thirst.

Any signs of fever in your pet may be the first indication of an infectious disease and I would advise you to consult a veterinary surgeon. Homoeopathic treatment may be used in conjunction with any antibiotics prescribed by the vet and is particularly helpful if virus infection is present.

Treatment

Aconite (Remedy 1): A few doses at fifteen to thirty minute intervals are indicated at the onset of fever.

Gelsemium (Remedy 12): Gelsemium may be used if the fever is not accompanied by increased thirst and there is obvious dullness and sleepiness. Shivering is also marked as in influenza. One tablet two hourly on the first day then one four times daily (four hourly) for three or four days until relief.

Sulphur (Remedy 22): Sulphur is useful in cases when there is a high temperature and virus infection is suspected. One tablet twice daily for up to three days should be sufficient.

Footnote
Homoeopathic doctors have a great number of remedies to choose from when treating fevers and the final selection depends very much on particular symptoms. We can and should wherever possible apply this 'fine tuning' approach to animals.

In addition to the three remedies outlined above, the veterinary pack contains several others that also have the ability to act in treating a fever.

Arsenic (Remedy 4): When there is a lot of sneezing, restlessness and a desire for warmth.

Apis mel (Remedy 2): Indicated when any sort of warmth seems to aggravate the condition.

Bryonia (Remedy 5): When there is much coughing, great thirst and feeling worse for moving about.

Rhus tox (Remedy 19): When there is coughing, weakness, prostration and yet restlessness and a wish to move about.

FITS – HYSTERIA – EPILEPSY

Fits are very distressing for the owner, especially the first time one occurs. If there is any suspicion that your pet may have suffered a fit then it is most important that you consult a veterinary surgeon.

The animal will usually begin by frothing at the mouth, occasionally vomiting beforehand, and it will then lie on its side paddling furiously with its front and hind legs. It often passes water and sometimes passes a motion as well. The fit may last as little as thirty seconds or go on for several minutes. After the fit the animal may appear dazed and dull for quite a while and in severe cases goes straight from one fit into another.

The reason why an animal suddenly has a fit is often obscure. A fit seems to be a sort of safety valve for the brain, rather like the steam escaping from a pressure cooker as it reaches its maximum pressure. Fits are more likely to occur in highly-strung nervous animals and are seldom seen in the placid pet.

Treatment
(after consulting your veterinary surgeon)

Cocculus (Remedy 9): One dose every four hours (or more often if necessary) may help to overcome this distressing condition.

Scutellaria (Remedy 20): For the hysterical type of very highly-strung pet that is likely to have a fit from sheer excitement. One tablet twice daily up to two or three days at a time if necessary.

FLATULENCE

The passing of wind sometimes accompanied by marked rumblings in the abdomen is commonplace in animals. It is not surprising when one thinks about the various extraordinary and often disgusting things that a dog, for instance, will eat or lick at. Cats, too, may eat mice, birds and small rabbits – fur and all – and these have got to either be vomited back or pass through the intestines which may have a considerable job to digest them! Wind is often the result.

Treatment

Carbo veg (Remedy 7): In acute cases where there is discomfort a tablet may be given every fifteen minutes until relief.

In the chronic case where it is more of a social problem I would advise a tablet one hour before a meal. Alternatively, give tablet with the first signs of trouble or try a course of tablets, giving one two or three times daily for a few days. This may stop the condition for a while at least.

Nux vomica (Remedy 17): Nux vomica is indicated when the flatulence is combined with digestive upsets resulting in diarrhoea which may last a day or two at a time. One tablet three times daily for a few days as necessary.

FLEAS

Fleas are a terrible problem in our domestic pets and seem to have been on the increase in recent years. They are dark brown in colour and their droppings which can be seen on the skin at the base of the hair look like coal-dust and are sometimes mistaken for this.

The life cycle of a flea is very short, less than a week, and it is therefore most important to treat with baths and dusting powders frequently in order to interrupt the life cycle and the production of eggs. Fleas have to get off the animal to breed and their eggs are laid in the bedding or about the house on the carpets or chairs, so these must be treated at the same time as you treat your pet.

Flea-bites do not seem to affect some animals and in fact some never seem to get bitten whilst others appear to be highly susceptible to the bites which cause severe irritation leading to much scratching and eczema.

Treatment

Apis (Remedy 2); *Arsenic* (Remedy 4); *Cantharis* (Remedy 6); *Merc sol* (Remedy 16); *Rhus tox* (Remedy 19); *Sulphur* (Remedy 22): These are all treatments for eczema and are dealt with in more detail under *Skin Conditions*.

Pulex → flea Norde

Footnote
It is possible to get a homoeopathic potency made of almost anything from house dust to sunlight and a potency of flea (Pulex) is available. Such a remedy could be useful where the flea-bites cause a really troublesome allergic reaction on the animal's skin (or the human's!).

FLU
(See *Influenza*)

FRACTURES
(See *Broken Bones*)

FRIGHT
(See *Fear*)

GUMS – GINGIVITIS

Inflamed gums are usually associated with the accumulation of tartar on the teeth, or with rotten teeth which are eroding the gums and setting up inflammation. Inflammation and infection of the gums is quite common in cats.

Treatment

Hepar sulph (Remedy 13): For infected gums that bleed easily with an offensive smell to the breath. One tablet three times daily.

Merc sol (Remedy 16): The best all-round remedy for gum

troubles, when the gums are receding, bleed easily, the teeth are loose and the breath is very offensive. Give one tablet every two to four hours (four to six daily) for a few days, while awaiting and after professional attention.

HAEMORRHAGE

Haemorrhage is the medical term for loss of blood from any of the blood-vessels of the body. The blood may flow externally as with a cut or injury, or there may be internal bleeding, for instance as with Warfarin rat poisoning which can be much more difficult to diagnose. See *Bleeding* for treatment.

HARDPAD

This is a variation of the disease caused by the distemper virus and not a separate viral infection as was at first thought. The crusty, peeling pads are one of the final symptoms to develop during the course of this long and distressing disease. See *Distemper* for more details and treatment.

HEART CONDITIONS

Any heart condition may be serious and must be investigated by your veterinary surgeon. The heart cough which is commonplace among middle-aged and older dogs, particularly those that tend to be overweight, can be treated quite successfully with homoeopathy. There are frequent bouts of a dry, harsh cough, finishing up with a retch as if the animal wished to bring something up, but seldom does.

Such a cough sounds terrible but is often more troublesome and worrying for the owner than for the dog itself.

Treatment

Spongia (Additional Remedy): One tablet three times daily for ten days. Repeat as required, but if there is little or no response other homoeopathic remedies are available through a veterinary surgeon who uses homoeopathy.

HEPATITIS

Hepatitis is an inflammation of the liver. A serious liver disease that occurs in dogs is called canine virus hepatitis (CVH) or Rubarth's disease and this is usually prevented by vaccination at the time that the puppy has his 'jabs' at six to twelve weeks of age. For this reason the condition is not seen frequently nowadays.

If a liver condition has been diagnosed in your dog the following remedies may be of some help, probably in conjunction with the use of ordinary medicines.

Treatment

Nux vomica (Remedy 17): For liver conditions and chronic bowel upsets for no obvious reason. One tablet four hourly for two to three days may help this condition.

Pulsatilla (Remedy 18): Pulsatilla can be useful if a liver condition has been confirmed. Two symptoms could point to the use of pulsatilla. The first is the vomiting of undigested food eaten some hours previously. The second is the changeable nature of the motion which is hard one day and soft or watery the next. There is usually no increased thirst in this type of liver involvement.

Alternative Remedy

Chelidonium (common celandine): This is a very good remedy for any ailment in which the liver is thought to be involved.

There is often much yawning, poor appetite and possibly jaundice present. One tablet every four hours (four daily), continued for a few days if there seems to be some improvement.

HICCUP

A common condition in young puppies that can sometimes be troublesome. We cannot ask our pets to hold their breath, or drink water backwards or any of the other traditional 'cures' that we use, including giving them a fright or suddenly making a loud noise which would be unkind.

Treatment

Nux vomica (Remedy 17): This is a wonderful remedy for any sort of digestive upset. Give one tablet immediately the hiccups start and repeat in half an hour if necessary.

HYSTERIA
(See *Fits*)

INCONTINENCE (Enuresis)

Inability to hold urine which is passed sometimes without the animal being aware of it. This is mainly a condition of the old and the very young. We all know of the old dog or cat who leaks in his bed or on the carpet without seeming to realize that it has happened. Likewise we can all visualize the excited little puppy rushing to greet us and tiddling with sheer joy and happiness. The above sorts of incontinence of the aged and the young can be difficult to treat but homoeopathic remedies are worth trying. Incontinence also takes place in some bitches when they are in season or when they are in whelp (in pup).

Treatment

Apis (Remedy 2): For the pet who is bursting and seems unable to wait until it can get outside. One tablet four times daily for three to four days. Repeat if helpful.

Merc cor (Remedy 15): Merc Cor is indicated where the animal appears to pass more than it has drunk, which is an observation I hear in the surgery from time to time. One tablet every four hours (four daily) for a few days.

Pulsatilla (Remedy 18): This may be given when your pet is pregnant or having a phantom or false pregnancy, or if there is incontinence when a bitch is in season. One tablet every four hours (four daily) for a few days.

Sulphur (Remedy 22): For incontinence and the frequent urge to pass urine, almost like cystitis. One tablet three times daily.

Alternative Remedy

Baryta carb: This is the remedy that we shall all come to eventually! It is the one that homoeopathic doctors use for senility or senile dementia, as it is known. This remedy is worth trying for incontinence in the very old and the very young. One tablet twice daily for a week and repeated perhaps a week or two later.

Footnote

Incontinence may be confused with cystitis and the remedies and symptoms of this condition are to be found under the heading *Cystitis*.

INDIGESTION

We do not know if animals suffer from heartburn but we do know that they quite frequently have digestive upsets (see also *Colic*). Vomiting after a meal and spasmodic bouts of diarrhoea for no apparent reason, or the after-effects of scavenging as in the case of dogs, or eating mice, birds or small rabbits in the case of cats may well cause indigestion which is hardly surprising (see also *Flatulence*).

Treatment

Nux Vomica (Remedy 17): This is the best remedy for any sort of digestive upset or over-indulgence in both animals and man. One tablet every two to four hours whenever and for as long as discomfort appears to persist.

INFLUENZA

Dogs: Flu as we know it in human beings rarely occurs in dogs but occasionally a dog becomes suddenly ill with a high temperature, loss of appetite, coughing, running eyes and sometimes stiffness in the back and other joints (see also *Fever*).

Treatment

Gelsemium (Remedy 12): One tablet every two hours on the first day then one four times daily (four hourly) for three or four days if necessary.

Cats: Cat flu is a well-recognized condition and is widespread among the cat population of Britain. On many farms, for instance, it is a persistent disease passing from generation to generation, with some weaker kittens unable to survive an attack, but others developing an immunity. This virus disease of cats has many similarities to human flu. The symptoms are streaming, watery eyes, much sneezing, stuffed-up nose, often with a crusty discharge round the nostrils, coughing and sometimes dribbling. There is usually loss of appetite and dullness.

Treatment

Aconite (Remedy 1): Aconite in the early stages – one tablet every hour for two to three hours.

Gelsemium (Remedy 12): One tablet every two hours during the first day and then continue four times daily for three to four days as long as the attack is a mild one and improvement is obvious.

Alternative Remedies

Allium cepa – a homoeopathic potency of onions is very helpful if watery eyes are the prevalent symptom.

Rhus tox (Remedy 19) is useful if there is a dry cough combined with the other symptoms.

Footnote
Severe and persistent cat flu requires treatment with antibiotics but the remedies outlined above can ease the symptoms and relieve the mild case.

Vaccination
Vaccination with nasal drops or by injection has been developed in the last few years and is very effective. I always recommend owners to have their cats vaccinated regularly, particularly if they go to boarding kennels or catteries.

A homoeopathic oral vaccine against feline influenza is also available if preferred but I have no experience with it.

INJURIES

Injuries can be of many and various types and I have described them under *Accidents, Bites, Bruises, Shock* and *Wounds*, or according to the place of the injury (e.g. eye).

Treatment

Aconite (Remedy 1): If there is any element of shock associated with the injury it is always worth giving a dose or two of aconite at fifteen to thirty minute intervals while the extent of the injury is being assessed and, if necessary, veterinary attention is being sought.

Arnica (Remedy 3): Arnica is absolutely the remedy of choice in any sort of injury that involves bruising, swelling and haemorrhage. Give one tablet every two hours up to four doses, then one three times daily as required.

JAUNDICE

The liver is one of the vital organs of our bodies and it produces a substance known as bile which aids the process of digestion. The bile in most animals (except the horse) is stored in the gall-bladder and flows down the bile duct into the duodenum or first part of the intestine, where it mixes with the foodstuffs as they pass down the alimentary canal (or bowels). This bile is greenish-yellow in colour and if for some reason its passage into the intestines is obstructed it circulates in the blood and the characteristic yellow colour of the skin and mucous membranes (inside the mouth and inner eyelids etc.) results.

Infectious jaundice (leptospiral jaundice of dogs) also causes Weil's disease in man. Weil's disease is carried by about 40-50 per cent of apparently healthy rats and their urine may contaminate human and animal food. It can cause a serious illness in man which fortunately nowadays can be treated successfully with antibiotics.

The disease is caused by a spirochaete (a type of bacteria which has a spiral or wavy outline. Incidently, syphilis, one of the venereal diseases of man, is caused by another spirochaete.) Two leptospiral diseases occur in dogs – leptospira ictero-haemorrhagiae, the one that causes the infectious disease mentioned above and leptospira canicola, which causes a kidney infection in the dog.

Both these conditions can be prevented by vaccination and are usually included in the puppy inoculations.

Treatment

Nux vomica (Remedy 17): One tablet every four hours for a few days until the jaundice begins to disappear. This remedy is useful in conditions where the jaundice is accompanied by other symptoms such as vomiting and alternating constipation and diarrhoea.

Alternative Remedy

Chelidonium majus (celandine): Chelidonium majus is probably the best remedy for the treatment of jaundice and liver complaints. One tablet every four hours (four daily) until the jaundice has disappeared.

KIDNEY DISEASE – NEPHRITIS

This is one of the most common conditions seen in both dogs and cats. The frequency of the occurrence of this condition in our pets is probably due in part to the fact that they like to eat protein foods (meat eaters) and one of the tests that we carry out on the urine of suspect cases is to see if protein is escaping via the kidneys into the urine. Excessive and sudden thirst is often one of the first symptoms that is noticeable in kidney disease.

Acute Nephritis

In cases of acute nephritis the animal is obviously ill. In addition to the thirst there is loss of appetite and vomiting. There may also be a temperature, dullness and an arched back which may be painful and dehydration soon follows.

Chronic Nephritis

Chronic nephritis develops in a good many elderly dogs and cats and is sadly one of the main causes of death in our household pets. There is usually thirst, some loss of appetite and vomiting, dullness and a gradual loss of weight in both cats and dogs. Eventually there is dehydration and tremors develop due to waste products normally passed out in the urine accumulating in the body, causing a condition known as uraemia. Ultimately uraemic convulsions and death will follow. Both acute and chronic nephritis require veterinary treatment.

Homoeopathic Treatment

Merc sol (Remedy 16):

Acute Nephritis: One tablet two hourly during the first day, then one four hourly (four daily) until the attack subsides.

Chronic Nephritis: One tablet four times daily (four hourly) for up to ten days. Repeat at regular intervals, at least monthly if a good response is achieved.

Cantharis (Remedy 6): Cantharis may be used if there is blood in the urine. One tablet every two hours during the first day, then every four hours (four daily) until relief.

LEPTOSPIROSIS

Leptospirosis occurs in two forms in dogs:

1. Leptospira icterohaemorrhagiae which causes jaundice in dogs and man (Weil's disease) is described under *Jaundice*.

2. Leptospira canicola is a more common infection in dogs, causing nephritis. This may be acute or subacute and the symptoms are variable. The main ones are loss of appetite, fever and dullness which may be accompanied by extreme

thirst, vomiting and loss of weight. There is a characteristic sickly-sweet odour to the body followed by twitchings and death.

Both forms of leptospirosis can be prevented by vaccination which is usually included in the puppy inoculations and the immunity is then maintained by annual booster injections. Homoeopathic oral vaccines against the two leptospiral infections are also available.

Treatment
Leptospira icterohaemorrhagiae – see *Jaundice*.
Leptospira canicola – see *Kidney Disease – Nephritis*.

LICE

Lice are small parasites that live and breed on the host animal. They are spread from one animal to another by direct contact or through bedding or occasionally grooming utensils. They appear as minute, grey objects crawling about at the base of the hair and they feed by sucking blood or biting their hosts. Different species occur on all our domestic animals. The eggs of the lice cling steadfastly to the hair, as anybody who has had a child at school with 'nits' (which are the eggs, not the lice) will know.

Treatment
This must first be aimed at getting rid of the lice themselves and this can be done using various proprietary preparations in the form of shampoos and dusting powders available from veterinary surgeons, pet supply shops and some health stores and chemists.
   The lice cause intense irritation and the only way the animal can try to get some relief is by scratching and rubbing, which in turn may cause soreness and eczema.
   See under *Skin Conditions* for the various remedies available in the veterinary pack for treating eczema etc.

MANGE

Mange is caused by tiny animals known as mites which live in the surface of the skin of the host animal and cause intense irritation. This may lead to almost continuous scratching in some cases. During the nineteenth century the condition scabies in man, caused by a mange mite, was commonplace and hence today we still use the word 'mangy' in everyday language as a descriptive term.

Treatment

Sulphur (Remedy 22): Sulphur is good for relieving the irritation of mange because of the heat produced in the skin by the burrowing mites. This irritation is made worse by the act of scratching and from any source of external heat. One tablet twice daily for four to five days and repeated after a couple of weeks if there is definite improvement.

Arsenic (Remedy 4): This is an alternative remedy that may be tried if the sulphur fails to give relief. One tablet four times daily for a few days.

Additional Remedy
Psorinum is a remedy that is prepared from the scabies mange vesicle. It has a deep-seated and lasting action and is therefore best used under the guidance of a homoeopath.

MASTITIS – MAMMITIS

Inflammation of the mammary glands is a common condition of milking cows and is also seen frequently in lactating goats, pigs and sheep. It is less commonly seen in mares, bitches and cats.

The mammary glands become hot, inflamed and painful and these symptoms may be accompanied by a high temperature, loss of appetite and depression (dullness).

Mastitis can occur in animals that are not lactating (producing milk) but is more usually seen in those giving milk. In domestic pets it is nearly always an acute mastitis that we have to deal with.

Treatment

Bryonia (Remedy 5): Bryonia is indicated when the glands are hot, painful and very hard. Other indications for choosing bryonia are if the animal keeps still and is obviously reluctant to move and also wants to lie on the cold floor away from any heat. One tablet every two hours on the first day, then four times daily (four hourly) until relief.

Chamomilla (Remedy 8): Chamomilla is the remedy for acute pain so is indicated if this is the main symptom of the mastitis. One tablet every fifteen to thirty minutes for a few doses if necessary, then every two to four hours.

Hepar sulph (Remedy 13): Useful when infection is present and the animal clings to the warmth (opposite of bryonia). One tablet three to four times daily according to the severity of the condition.

Pulsatilla (Remedy 18): This remedy is usually associated with females and suits the quiet, placid animal with the inflammation seen in phantom pregnancy (see *False Pregnancy*). Give one tablet three to four times daily for a few days.

Alternative Remedy

Phytolacca: This is the all-purpose remedy for mastitis which may be tried with any or all the symptoms described above. One tablet three to four times daily for a few days.

Footnote

Here again (compare *Fever*) we have a number of remedies to choose from and careful observation of the main symptoms is important in making the correct choice. If in any doubt seek professional advice.

METRITIS – PYOMETRA

Metritis is an inflammation of the uterus (womb) usually associated with an infection. It occurs quite commonly in bitches, less so in queens (female cats), but may be seen in any animal.

This is a condition which requires urgent veterinary attention. The symptoms often appear soon (within a few weeks) after the season and are thirst, inappetence, extreme dullness or lethargy, possibly a temperature and some swelling of the abdomen. There may or may not be a discharge from the vulva.

Treatment
(in addition to veterinary attention which may include surgery to remove the womb)

The Acute Case: Surgery is usually the outcome of acute metritis or pyometra (infection in the womb), as it is commonly known.

Arnica (Remedy 3): Give arnica every two to four hours before and after any surgical operation. It will help to counteract any shock, reduce haemorrhage and ease bruising and pain.

The Chronic Case: The slight discharge with few other symptoms, occasionally seen in the older animal.

Arsenic (Remedy 4): This remedy helps the sluggish, tired, soon-exhausted bitch with a uterine discharge and great thirst. One tablet four times daily for a few days.

Alternative Remedy
Sepia and Sabina are other remedies that seem to help the chronic type of metritis. One tablet three times daily until the

discharge ceases and the animal appears to feel better.

NAILS

I mention nails because broken, split and mis-shapen nails are seen in our pets (and ourselves) and can be a nuisance, causing some lameness and discomfort.

Treatment

Silica (Remedy 21): One tablet twice daily for two to three weeks may be necessary to improve the quality of the nail as it grows.

NAUSEA
(See *Vomiting*)

NEPHRITIS
(See *Kidney Disease*)

NERVOUS CONDITIONS

The nervy, excitable, highly-strung dog is seen too often nowadays in my opinion and I am afraid some of this type of 'temperament' must be due to close or in-breeding. Such breeding is designed to bring out good points of conformation (shape) with too little regard for the 'nature' of the animal that is the result.

Treatment

Scutellaria (Remedy 20): This is a remedy that I have found useful in treating unruly behaviour, overexcitability and destructiveness particularly in younger dogs (juvenile delinquents!) when they are left alone and become bored. It also seems to suit highly-bred cats of uncertain temperament.

Give one tablet twice daily for up to a week and then stop treatment to assess results. (On one occasion one tablet seemed to make the dog far worse, but on ceasing treatment no further trouble or destructiveness was encountered.) Treatment may be repeated when necessary if it appears to be beneficial.

Footnote

One case I remember well was an Irish setter pup of about six months who hated to be left without human company, although there was always an older setter in the house with him. Systematically he pulled all the books off the shelves that he could reach and tore them to pieces and when his owner returned he would be lying curled up in the bath! A few doses of scutellaria soon put him right and he is now a reformed character.

Chorea – St Vitus's Dance

This is a nervous condition in which there are involuntary jerking movements of one of the limbs and sometimes the head. The movements are irregular, being more marked sometimes, particularly if the animal is tired and they also may occur when the affected animal is resting or sleeping. If a dog survives an attack of distemper it may be left with chorea if the virus which eventually enters the brain damages part of it permanently.

Treatment

Causticum (Potassium hydroxide): One tablet once or twice daily for up to ten days may help to relieve this tiring condition. If it appears to help it may be repeated about once a month.

Conium maculatum (Common hemlock): This remedy helps if there is a progressive weakness of the hind legs seen usually in

the heavier breeds as they get older. One tablet three times daily
for ten days. Repeat in two to three months if it appears to help
the condition.

NOSE
(See also *Catarrh* and *Sinusitis*)

Bleeding from the nose occurs in both dogs and cats and
occasionally in other animals. It occurs quite frequently in
horses – particularly racehorses – when they are fit (epistaxis).
Nosebleeds may be spontaneous but are more often the result of
a blow or knock on the nose which damages and bruises the
delicate coiled bones inside the nostril.

Treatment

Arnica (Remedy 3): For the steady trickle of blood from the
nostril associated with bruising and haemorrhage, probably
from an injury of some sort. One tablet every hour up to four
doses, followed by one three to four times daily for as long as
necessary.

Sneezing
Sneezing may be apparent in any animal and is often associated
with influenza in the cat and various allergies in the other
species.

Treatment

Arsenic (Remedy 4); *Gelsemium* (Remedy 12): For sneezing
bouts with no apparent cause try one of the above remedies.
Give one tablet hourly up to four, then one four hourly if
necessary. See also *Influenza – Cat Flu*.

OPERATIONS

Homoeopathy is strongly indicated and of great benefit before and after any operation (including dental treatment).

Treatment

Arnica (Remedy 3): Give one tablet four times daily (every four hours) for two or three days before a routine operation and after any operation repeat for seven to ten days if necessary. This will help to control shock, haemorrhage and bruising.

PAIN

Animals obviously suffer pain in much the same way as we do ourselves, but the difficulty is to assess the degree of pain involved and sometimes also the part of the body that is painful.

Acute Pain
Symptoms: restlessness, panting or sweating, obvious discomfort, sometimes – as in colic – the animal looks round at its side or kicks at its abdomen with a hind leg. In extreme pain the animal will throw itself on the ground and writhe about and may cry out or groan (see *Colic*). There is usually no appetite and depending on the reason for the pain, there may be vomiting and diarrhoea.

Treatment

Hypericum (Remedy 14): Hypericum is helpful for injuries involving feet and nails, and any general unspecified painful condition. One tablet every two to four hours if relief is apparent.

Chamomilla (Remedy 8): This is a remedy for the sudden acute pain seen in such conditions as toothache, earache or the acute muscular pain of a sudden back injury or pulled muscle, etc.

Give a tablet as often as necessary (five to fifteen minutes). A response should be apparent within an hour of commencing treatment. Continue two to four hourly if necessary.

Chronic Pain

This is the slow, nagging kind of pain that we experience with a long-standing ailment such as backache or rheumatism, or after an accident or injury.

To obtain relief from chronic pain it is particularly important to relate the remedy to the symptoms presented.

Animals with slight or chronic pain usually continue to eat and behave much as usual but are obviously not quite themselves.

Treatment
Related to symptoms presented; for example:

symptoms of colic – *Colocynth* (Remedy 10);
symptoms of pain in feet – *Hypericum* (Remedy 14);
pain in muscle joints – *Rhus tox* (Remedy 19);
toothache; rubbing mouth; teeth rotten, etc. – *Chamomilla* (Remedy 8).

Footnote
Remember that pain is a protective mechanism telling us and our pets to take care and not to overdo it after a strain or injury, etc. We cannot tell our pets to have a cup of tea and take an aspirin and stay in bed, so as soon as they feel better they will tend to rush around and over-exert themselves too quickly, which may lead to a disappointing relapse.

This is why corticosteroids, anti-inflammatory agents and muscle relaxants, etc. can sometimes do more harm than good. They simply remove the pain but not the reason for it and the animal feels better and overdoes things. It is up to us, the owners of our pets, to be watchful and control them until we are quite sure that a cure has been achieved.

PANIC
(See *Fear*)

PARALYSIS

Paralysis may be the result of an accident or an injury or be due to damage to part of the brain (from a stroke, for instance).

Hemiplegia
Paralysis of one side of the body. This happens quite often to humans after a stroke, but is fortunately less common in animals and if it does occur it is usually a partial paralysis rather than a total one which would be impractical to treat. The animal with partial paralysis will tend to stagger sideways or even fall over as it walks, it may circle continuously in one direction and frequently holds its head down to one side. After recovery, which fortunately often follows a stroke, the head may be held noticeably to one side when the animal becomes tired.

Paraplegia (including 'Slipped Disc')
Paralysis of the back legs and rear part of the body. Total paraplegia is difficult to treat in animals because there may well be involuntary passing of urine or faeces (motions) or alternatively a complete cessation of these natural functions.

Paraplegia due to an accident will start to resolve quite quickly if it is only caused by bruising, swelling and pressure on the affected nerves. If no improvement is seen after a few days it is likely that there has been permanent damage either to the spine or the brain. Your veterinary surgeon will be able to advise you on the extent of the damage and the likely outcome of the case.

Treatment

Arnica (Remedy 3): If the paralysis is due to any sort of accident or injury, a few doses of arnica at hourly intervals on the first day can be helpful. Afterwards the arnica may be continued four times daily and, if desired, at the same time a second more specific remedy given.

Additional Remedies

Conium maculatum (Common hemlock): One tablet three times daily for ten days, repeated in two to four months if a response is achieved.

Causticum (for older animals): One tablet once or twice daily for up to ten days. Repeat each month if it appears to be helpful.

Hypericum (Remedy 14): One tablet every two to four hours can help to ease any pain or discomfort associated with the paralysis.

PARTURITION
(See *Birth*)

PARVOVIRUS DISEASE

Canine Parvovirus is a new disease of dogs that first appeared in many different parts of the world in 1978.

In young puppies under five weeks old it affects the heart muscle causing heart failure, weakness, collapse and death. Those puppies that survive this initial attack are left with weakened hearts and frequently die a few weeks or months later. In older puppies and adult dogs the virus causes severe vomiting and diarrhoea with rapid dehydration, soon followed by collapse and death.

Immediate veterinary attention should be sought if Parvovirus disease is suspected, when fluid therapy in the form of a drip given into the bloodstream may be tried. Unfortunately many cases do not respond to treatment and prevention should be the aim of every dog owner.

Treatment

Merc Cor (Remedy 15) or *Arsenic* (Remedy 4) may be tried in conjunction with ordinary medicine if there seems to be any chance of survival. These two remedies are both very useful in the treatment of acute vomiting and diarrhoea (see under list of remedies towards the end of the book for dosage etc.).

Vaccination

Vaccinations against Parvovirus disease are now freely available and effective. It is also possible to use a homoeopathic oral vaccine if this is preferred, but I have no experience of this preparation.

PINING

Occasionally we come across dogs that just cannot bear to be parted from their owners and cry piteously when they are left alone.

Treatment

Pulsatilla (Remedy 18): This is for the dog that barks continuously when it is left alone in the house. One dose twice daily for two or three days each month may help to resolve this problem.

Additional Remedy

Ignatia: In humans this is the remedy used for grief, for instance, after the death of a relative or friend. It can also be used for the pet who is pining because its owner is away. Give one tablet three times daily for up to one week if a response is achieved.

PNEUMONIA

Pneumonia is an inflammation of the lungs. There are many

different types of pneumonia but the one concerned with in animals are those caused by viruses or bacteria. Pneumonia is one of the last events that may occur after an infection enters the nose. The first line of defence against such infections tonsils and other glands at the back of the mouth in the region of the throat. Once past these glands the infection proceeds down the windpipe (trachea) and into the hollow tubes that supply the lungs with air – the bronchi – hence bronchitis. Finally the inflammation and infection reach the lung tissue itself, causing pneumonia. If the outer covering of the lungs which is in contact with the chest wall becomes involved too, we get pleurisy.

Symptoms

Heavy or increased rate of breathing, panting and in extreme cases a bluish tinge to the inner side of the lips, the gums and the tongue will develop as the tissues become starved of oxygen. Collapse and death may soon follow if treatment is not started immediately. Pneumonia in the dog is a very serious, often fatal, condition but fortunately, is not all that common. The characteristic symptom is a billowing or puffing out of the lips as the dog breathes out and this may be accompanied by a hissing noise.

Cats also suffer from pneumonia, particularly those that will stay out all night, whatever the weather, and then curl up in the hottest place in the house and get overheated. Cats with pneumonia are restless and tend to sit up with their mouths open as they pant for breath.

If pneumonia is suspected consult a veterinary surgeon as soon as possible.

Treatment

Aconite (Remedy 1): A few doses at half-hourly intervals (up to four) at the onset of any fever, including pneumonia, can be helpful.

Bryonia (Remedy 5): Bryonia is indicated when any sort of

movement – even that of breathing – seems to cause discomfort or pain. One tablet every four hours for several days.

Sulphur (Remedy 22): Sulphur may be used when the animal seems excessively hot, has a persistent cough and a thick, yellow discharge, which is frequently spat out. One tablet twice daily for up to five days.

PREGNANCY

Once pregnancy has been established or is suspected, the remedy Caulophyllum can be given during the three or four weeks before parturition (birth).

One tablet of potency twelve or potency thirty given daily will ease the discomfort sometimes experienced during labour. See also *Birth*.

Agalactia
(Milk absent or scarce). This is a condition seen soon after the young are born and is serious if the offspring are not to perish from starvation and dehydration.

Treatment

Pulsatilla (Remedy 18): A few doses of pulsatilla while the labour is taking place can help to calm the animal, ease the birth process and promote the production of milk. One tablet every half an hour.

Urtica (Remedy 24): One or two tablets given two hours apart may help to stimulate the milk to flow.

Footnote
It is most important that every new-born arrival suckles from its mother within a few hours of birth to obtain the first milk (colostrum) which is rich in nutrients and antibodies which give vital protection against many diseases.

PYOMETRA

Pyometra is an infection of the womb (uterus) when it becomes filled with poison. There may or may not be a discharge from the vulva. This condition frequently develops within a few weeks of the end of a season and is often accompanied by greatly increased thirst, loss of appetite, dullness and a general loss of interest in going for walks, etc. If this condition is suspected see a veterinary surgeon as soon as possible because it can be serious.

Treatment
See *Metritis*.

RHEUMATISM

A general definition of the word rheumatism could be 'pain and stiffness in joint and muscles'. I have dealt with the inflammation of joints under *Arthritis* so I will confine this section to dealing with muscular rheumatism.

Acute Rheumatism
I use this term to describe a condition seen usually in sporting dogs or those that suddenly take excessive exercise when they are not really fit for it.

There is a marked stiffening of the muscles of the back (lumbago) and often of the hind legs too, occasionally the front limbs are involved as well. On the day after the exercise the animal is very reluctant to move at all and if encouraged to do so may appear to have paralysis of the hind legs and be unable to stand up, certainly without assistance. Once on their feet they ease a little as they begin to move, but are still very stiff and obviously in a good deal of discomfort.

Treatment

Rhus tox (Remedy 19): One tablet every two hours up to four tablets, then one four times daily for a day or two until the condition eases.

Bryonia (Remedy 5): This is indicated in the few cases seen in the younger animal where the lameness appears to get worse with movement or exercise. Give one tablet four times daily until relief.

Chronic Rheumatism

This is a difficult condition to treat successfully with ordinary medicine or homoeopathy, but a number of remedies are worth trying and the one selected depends on the symptoms presented. The stiffness and pains of chronic rheumatism tend to recur frequently or appear to be more or less permanent.

Treatment

Rhus tox (Remedy 19): Try Rhus tox if there is any sort of easing of the stiffness or lameness as the animal begins to move about. One tablet every four hours for as long as necessary if any relief is observed.

Bryonia (Remedy 5): If the condition worsens with movement. One tablet every four hours until relief.

Sulphur (Remedy 22): When there is general stiffness and other remedies do not seem to help, trying a few doses of sulphur may produce the desired effect. Give one tablet twice daily for up to a week if some relief seems to be the result. Do not repeat too often (for at least two to three weeks).

Additional Remedy

Ruta: Ruta may be tried if the tendons and muscles appear to be involved in the condition. Give one tablet every four hours (four daily) until relief.

RINGWORM

This is a skin disease seen more often in country districts where farm animals frequently suffer from ringworm which may spread by contact to dogs and cats, etc. Circular, rather damp, areas of skin appear as the hair becomes damaged and falls out. Ringworm can easily spread to humans, especially from infected pets to children who fondle and kiss them and generally come into close contact with them. Ringworm is therefore a contagious disease, that is, it is spread by touch, and so care in handling infected animals and cleanliness are important to lower the risk of spread. If ringworm is suspected, a visit to the veterinary surgeon is advisable.

Homoeopathic Remedy

Tellurium: One tablet twice daily for seven to ten days can help to control this troublesome skin condition.

SCALDS

The difficulty with scalds and burns is that immediately after the incident the extent of the injury may be hidden by the hair. After a while this dead hair will fall out and a large wound may be revealed. If there is any doubt about the size of the burn or scald seek professional help.

Treatment

Aconite (Remedy 1): Give an aconite tablet immediately because there is bound to be some shock with such an injury.
    See *Burns* for other remedies.

SCRATCHING
(See *Skin Conditions*)

SENILITY

Senility is a state of mind that we see in aged and sometimes not that elderly people! Senility also occurs to an extent in dogs and cats. They seem confused and will wander aimlessly around the house, stand with their head in the corner for a while or perhaps begin to lose some control of their waterworks or bowels. It is almost as if they have not realized that they have spent a penny indoors, instead of in the garden where they have always gone in their younger days. I have known cats who will go out through the cat flap only to appear on the window sill a few minutes later asking to be let in, just so that they can repeat the process almost at once. In other respects such animals appear normal, eat their food hungrily and still enjoy life in their own way.

Treatment
A few doses of Baryta carb given three times daily for three or four days and repeated frequently may help.

SEPTICAEMIA

Septicaemia sometimes follows an infection with bacteria or viruses and is due to a poisoning of the whole body system. In the early stages there is usually a high temperature, extreme dullness, loss of appetite and increased thirst. This is a serious condition that would need a veterinary diagnosis and treatment.

Treatment

Aconite (Remedy 1): In the early stages three or four tablets given at fifteen to thirty minute intervals.

Arsenic (Remedy 4): Arsenic is useful if there is restlessness, vomiting and diarrhoea in addition to the symptoms mentioned earlier. Arsenic has the ability to make the patient (human or animal) feel better. One tablet every hour on the first day then one four times daily for two or three days.

Rhus tox (Remedy 19): If the septicaemia is accompanied by stiffness of muscles and joints, then Rhus tox can ease the discomfort and increase the animal's feeling of well-being. One tablet four times daily for a few days until relief.

Footnote
Homoeopathic remedies as I have said can be made from almost anything and a homoeopath may decide to use a remedy called pyrogen to treat septicaemia. This is made from putrifying lean beef that has been exposed to sunlight for some time and then potentized, and makes an invaluable remedy for some septic conditions!

In 1982 a farmer's wife who was looking after a number of orphan lambs caught 'Orf' on her finger. Orf is a particularly nasty and very contagious viral skin disease of sheep which occasionally infects humans and may be difficult to cure with ordinary medicine. The finger was very swollen, tender and red-looking, with an intense, throbbing pain. The lady told me that she was far too busy looking after all her lambs and bottle-feeing them to go and sit in the doctor's waiting room for hours and asked me to prescribe some homoeopathy. Treatment with pyrogen cleared the condition within a few days; the first dose brought relief from the painful throbbing in a few hours and there was no need to worry the doctor.

SHOCK

Shock to a varying degree accompanies any accident, injury or wound. It is quite safe and advisable to treat any such incident with a shock remedy and it is something positive that can be done while professional help is being summoned if it is necessary.

Treatment

Aconite (Remedy 1): This is the first remedy that comes to mind in any case where shock is involved. Give one tablet every quarter of an hour until calm is restored and any other treatment is under way.

Arnica (Remedy 3): This is another very useful remedy and can follow aconite in cases where there is bruising, haemorrhage and damage to tissues as well as the shock. One tablet every two hours on the first day, then one four times daily for a few days as necessary.

Carbo Veg (Remedy 7): This remedy is indicated only if there is a state of collapse with a bluish colour to the tongue, lips, etc. and the animal is unable to stand or does not seem fully conscious. One tablet every fifteen minutes, placed in the animal's mouth under the tongue, or crushed and the powder put onto the tongue, whilst awaiting veterinary attention.

SINUSITIS
(See also *Catarrh*)

Sinuses are hollow cavities in the bones of the head. The sinusus connect with the nose and sinusitis occurs if the lining of these cavities becomes inflamed and the hole filled with discharge (catarrh).

Treatment
See *Catarrh*.

Hepar Sulph (Remedy 13): In addition to the catarrh remedies this one may be useful if there is acute infection in the sinuses with a thick discharge which smells offensive. One tablet three times daily for four to five days.

SKIN CONDITIONS

Skin conditions of various kinds cause more troubles in our household pets than just about everything else put together. The reasons for these troubles may be obscure and complicated and range from simple parasitic infestations (fleas), to deep-seated and unknown allergies, and the many forms of eczema or dermatitis of nervous origin. In a book of this kind it is impossible to go into too much detail and I can only scratch the surface (please excuse the pun) of this vast subject. Acute or persistent skin complaints should be investigated by your veterinary surgeon, but homoeopathy can help to relieve some of the symptoms. Unfortunately many skin conditions are treated with corticosteroids and these preparations interfere with the action of our homoeopathic remedies. Do not be disappointed, therefore, if there is a poor response to your homoeopathic treatment, either if your pet has been taking any form of cortisone, or if the condition appears to be a complicated one. It seems to be difficult in many cases to pick the right remedy. The wrong remedy will do no harm but it will give little or no relief.

Eczema

Wet Eczema
Acute wet eczema can develop very quickly and is often a self-inflicted condition. Some incident (a flea-bite or wasp sting) irritates a part of the animal's skin which it then scratches, rubs, bites and licks vigorously until the hair has all been removed, leaving a bare, sticky, wet-looking patch of skin, which is extremely sensitive to the touch.

Treatment
I always remove a little hair from around the patch of eczema

...ms to tickle and stick to the area, aggravating the

Me..... . Remedy 16): Give a tablet every two hours on the first day (up to six) and then one four times daily for a few days. This remedy will work quickly if it is going to help and the affected area will begin to dry up within twenty-four hours and your pet will be paying less attention as time passes. If this is not the result you must get professional help which I would advise in any instance where the patch of eczema is larger than a ten-penny piece and getting bigger.

Additional Remedy

Croton tiglium: Croton tiglium is also effective in some cases of wet eczema, particularly in the outer part of the ear or in the region of the groin or genitals. One tablet every two hours up to six, then one four times daily for a few days.

Acute Dry Eczema

Acute dry eczema usually takes a little longer to develop so it is less dramatic but can cause as much irritation and scratching, etc. The hair may or may not be removed by the animal with dry eczema, but there are often red or raised, sometimes scaly, areas at the base of the hair.

Treatment

Sulphur (Remedy 22): Sulphur may be indicated if the skin is noticeably warm and dry and there is much itching. One tablet twice daily for a few days.

Chronic Eczema

This is a persistent condition which sometimes seems almost impossible to resolve. It may follow an acute attack or come on slowly due probably to some internal reaction (e.g. an allergy) or a psychological problem of some sort. This could be a change of owner, a change in the diet, change of circumstances – for instance, going to boarding kennels, or being parted from the owner for some reason.

Treatment

Arsenic (Remedy 4): Arsenic for dry, rough, scaly eczema with intense itching and sometimes inflammation and swelling of the affected area. One tablet three times daily for two days, followed by another two days' treatment a few days later if improvement is noticeable.

Rhus tox (Remedy 19): Rhus tox may be helpful if the condition starts as little blisters which soon rupture when the animal bites or scratches them. One tablet four times daily for a few days.

Sulphur (Remedy 22): Sulphur is a useful, all-round remedy and in chronic skin complaints may be given twice daily for two days to clear the system before following with another remedy.

Apis mel (Remedy 2): This can help in the type of acute eczema which follows a sting or insect bite. There will be intense reddening of the area which is sensitive and there may be some swelling and a blotchy appearance. Give one tablet four times daily for two to three days.

Cantharis (Remedy 6): This also has an effect on the skin and may be used if little blisters or vesicles with an angry, red look suddenly appear, particularly in the region of the genital organs. Cantharis is particularly useful in the treatment of burns or scalds. One tablet every hour up to four doses, then one four times daily for two to three days.

Urtica (Remedy 24): Urtica can also exert an action on the skin and might be selected for the acute allergic type of eczema, when there is marked irritation and an apparently stinging sensation which is obviously driving the animal to distraction. One tablet every hour or two in the really acute case, followed by one three times daily for two or three days.

Additional Remedy

Graphites is useful for the chronic wet eczema case which is seen less often but has thick, dry skin with cracks in it, which ooze a sticky, watery discharge, particularly seen in older, overweight animals.

Footnote

It is apparent, therefore, that many of the remedies in the veterinary pack have an action on the skin and any one might be selected to treat a case of eczema. In addition, there are dozens of other remedies that act on the skin, so it really is a matter of skill and attention to detail to select the correct one and achieve a response.

Dandruff – Scurf

Dandruff is the production of scales which are usually dry and flake-like. The scurf may be confined to the region of the back or be produced more or less all over the body. There may or may not be irritation with dandruff.

Treatment

Arsenic (Remedy 4): One tablet three times daily for three or four days and then wait for at least a week to see if the condition lessens.

Sulphur (Remedy 22): Sulphur is another very good general skin remedy and is indicated if the dandruff production is accompanied by much scratching. One tablet twice daily for three or four days, then cease treatment and assess results.

Dermatitis

This is an inflammation of the surface layers of the skin which may become infected if the animal scratches the area and damages the tissues. There may be pimple-like eruptions and the area is very sore and sensitive to touch.

Treatment

Hepar sulph (Remedy 13): One tablet three times daily for up to a week if necessary.

Itching and Scratching

It is quite normal for an animal to sit down and have a good scratch at some part of its body two or three times daily; we do it ourselves! However, persistent scratching indicates some underlying problem which may well be due to parasitic infection (fleas or lice) or may be due to an allergic reaction of some kind. The remedies that may be useful if there is much irritation and scratching will be found under the various headings *Eczema, Allergies, Stings*, etc.

Footnote

Remember many skin conditions are an outward manifestation or sign of an underlying problem which may well be of an allergic or a nervous nature.

A chronic long-standing skin complaint may take a long time to respond to homoeopathy because the remedy has to work from within the body, which takes time. There is no point, therefore, in persisting with a remedy for days on end. Give a few doses as directed and then wait at least a week to see if there is any response. If there is some improvement the remedy may be repeated in two to three weeks.

There are literally dozens of remedies available that have the facility to act on the skin and it is often extremely difficult to find the correct one. Homoeopaths will often dig deep into the individual's history, likes and dislikes, etc. before coming up with that particular person's constitutional or specific remedy that has the power to act on the whole body and reach the skin in that way. This is a more difficult approach to adopt with animals because we can only assess their symptoms and peculiarities by observation, but nevertheless it is a way which a homoeopathic veterinary surgeon may well wish to explore in tackling a skin problem.

SLIPPED DISC

This is a term that is loosely used to describe many conditions of the back, when a variable degree of pain and paralysis are present. Strictly speaking, the term should be confined to cases where an X-ray shows that one or more of the pads of cartilage (gristle) which lie between the bones in the back (the vertebrae) have ruptured or prolapsed, causing pressure on the spinal nerve which is running down inside the vertebrae.

Veterinary treatment is required for this condition which may well be serious.

Homoeopathic Treatment
See also *Paralysis – Paraplegia*

Nux vomica (Remedy 17): Nux vomica is useful in the acute case when there is pain, some paralysis and very tense, hard, back muscles that are in spasm. One tablet three times daily until relief.

SNAKE BITES

Snakebites occur quite commonly in some parts of the country. On very hot, sunny days snakes like to come out from the bushes etc. and bask in the sunshine. It is then that the dog may suddenly come upon them and either not be able to retreat in time or may deliberately investigate and get bitten.

The area that has been bitten, usually the mouth region or one of the feet, will swell up almost immediately to a large size, become very hard and cause marked discomfort and distress. Veterinary attention is required immediately.

Treatment
Homoeopathic treatment may be useful too.

Aconite (Remedy 1): A few doses of aconite given every fifteen minutes will help to relieve the shock which is always present with a snakebite. Snakebites naturally alarm the owner as well as the animal involved, so take a dose or two of aconite at the same time as you treat your pet!

Arnica (Remedy 3): After three or four doses of aconite, follow with arnica. Arnica will help to reduce the extreme swelling and bruising of the part of the body that has been bitten. One tablet every four hours (four daily) until relief.

SNEEZING

Sneezing may be associated with an allergy of some kind, an irritation of the nose from various dusts etc. and is a common symptom in cat flu.

Treatment

Gelsemium (Remedy 12): For sneezing when the cause is unknown. One tablet hourly up to four, then one four-hourly if required.

Arsenic (Remedy 4): Arsenic is another useful remedy for much sneezing. One tablet every hour up to four if necessary should be sufficient.

SPRAINS AND STRAINS

A sprain may be defined as the wrenching or twisting of a joint (e.g. sprained wrist or ankle) when there is some damage to its attachment.

A strain may mean much the same as a sprain, but is applied more to the over-exercise or over-exertion of muscles and tendons.

): Arnica may be used for any condition when
bruising or pain. One tablet three or four times
ef.

Rhus t Remedy 19): One tablet four times daily until relief
in any sprain or strain which seems to ease even slightly as the
animal begins to move about.

Symphytum (Remedy 23): This remedy, which is useful in
aiding the repair of fractures, may also help in cases of severe
strain involving the attachment of tendons and ligaments to the
bones. One tablet three times daily for seven to ten days if
improvement is taking place.

STINGS

Stings from bees, wasps and other insects can be troublesome to
animals, particularly puppies, who seem to love to try and catch
bees and wasps in their mouths and sometimes swallow them.

Treatment

Apis mel (Remedy 2): This is a remedy prepared from the bee
and on the 'like treats like' basis is definitely indicated for stings
of any sort. Give one tablet immediately and repeat in half an
hour if necessary. Treatment may be continued at hourly
intervals for the rest of the day if relief and reduction of any
swelling that may have occurred is obviously taking place.

Cantharis (Remedy 6): If the sting or insect bite is very
inflamed, red and angry-looking, give several doses of this
remedy at two-hourly intervals until relief.

STROKES

A stroke is a sudden attack of paralysis resulting from an injury to the brain or spinal cord. This damage is often caused by a small blood clot which lodges in the brain or spinal cord, exerting pressure on the nerves to some part of the body.

Treatment
See *Paralysis – Hemiplegia.*

SURGERY – SURGICAL OPERATIONS

There is a wonderful homoeopathic remedy that can be used before and after any operation, including dental treatment. This remedy helps to counteract shock, to control haemorrhage and reduces swelling and bruising.

Treatment

Arnica (Remedy 3): Arnica can be given for a few days before any routine operation and again after all surgery routine or emergency. Give one tablet every four hours for two or three days before the operation. Afterwards, if necessary, it can be repeated every two hours on the first day, then four times daily for a few days until recovery takes place.

TEETH
(See *Bad Breath* and *Gums*)

Teeth in older dogs and cats frequently go bad or collect large deposits of tartar which in turn erodes the gums and sets up infection. Teeth scaling and extractions, if necessary, can be done by your veterinary surgeon who includes dentistry with his other surgical skills. Dogs and cats living in today's society where they mostly eat prepared or tinned food can manage quite happily without any teeth, should they all have to be removed because of decay. The gums soon harden up and they seldom have problems eating their food, which they chew little in any case.

Teething
Young dogs and cats change their teeth around six months of age when the permanent teeth come into use. It is unusual for any troubles to arise at this time but if there is any soreness or apparent discomfort (rubbing the side of the mouth along the floor or scratching at the side of the mouth with a front paw), then there is a homoeopathic remedy which is used for humans with excellent results.

Treatment
Chamomilla (Remedy 8): Give a tablet every hour if necessary for a few doses and continue three or four times daily until relief.

THIRST

Some animals, like some people, drink more than others, which is of no consequence. It is a sudden change in drinking patterns or the amount drunk that is important to note. Sudden excessive thirst could be due to a fever, kidney disease, diabetes, pyometra in the female, or a number of other conditions. Conversely, an animal that ceases to drink at all soon becomes dehydrated, which may also be serious. Therefore any change in drinking habits which continues for more than a day or two should be investigated by your veterinary surgeon.

Footnote
On the 'like for like' principle I have occasionally treated excessive thirst successfully with homoeopathic doses of common salt!

TONSILLITIS

People often seem surprised to think that their pets have tonsils and are quite amazed when a diagnosis of tonsillitis is made by the vet.

Acute tonsillitis responds well to antibiotics which can soon remove the infection. However, recurrent tonsillitis in an animal causes chronic inflammation and swelling of the tonsils, as is commonly the case with children, too. This leads to a troublesome cough and it is in these chronic cases that homoeopathy can help to give relief.

Treatment

Hepar sulph (Remedy 13): Give one dose four times daily for a few days. It may be that a different potency is required to achieve good and lasting results, so seek professional help if necessary.

TRAVEL SICKNESS
(See *Car Sickness*)

URINARY DISORDERS
(See *Cystitis* and *Kidney Disease*)

URTICARIA (Nettle rash)

Urticaria is the sudden appearance of swellings in the head region or other parts of the body. Urticaria is a type of allergy and is therefore dealt with in more detail under the heading *Allergies*.

Treatment

Urtica (Remedy 24): One tablet every hour, up to four if necessary, followed by one four times daily until the swellings subside. These should disappear in twenty-four to thirty-six hours.

UTERINE DISORDERS
(See *Metritis* and *Pyometra*)

VACCINATION

Ordinary vaccines have been produced for some diseases for many years and new ones are being developed all the time. I would advise you, whatever sort of pet you own, to consult your veterinary surgeon about the various vaccines that are available for any animal, from a horse to a rabbit.

Homoeopathic oral vaccines are also produced for a number of common diseases but I have no experience of their use, although I have no reason to believe that they are not effective.

Vaccination Reactions

Occasionally an animal becomes ill after being vaccinated and if this does happen you should advise your veterinary surgeon as soon as possible.

A homoeopathic remedy called Thuja has been used for many years by homoeopathic doctors for the ill-effects of vaccination in humans. This remedy may also be used under the guidance of a homoeopathic veterinary surgeon for animals suffering some reaction following vaccination.

VOMITING (Sickness – Retching)

Vomiting does not seem to distress dogs or cats as much as it does most humans. Indeed many animals will proceed to eat their vomit (or somebody else's!) as soon as they have thrown up. Dogs and cats will sometimes eat rough grass in order to vomit, usually saliva or bile come up with the grass, almost as if they had decided to take a dose of medicine to make themselves sick. Therefore occasional vomiting, particularly in view of the extraordinary things that animals eat, is nothing to worry about. Repeated vomiting on the other hand may be serious and is always noteworthy. If a remedy is going to work it will usually act quickly, so if vomiting persists or is happening more frequently in spite of the remedy that you have given, seek veterinary advice.

Treatment

Arsenic (Remedy 4): The animal is often thirsty and vomits the water back almost immediately after having a drink. Vomiting may occur several times in the space of one or two hours or there may be almost simultaneous vomiting and diarrhoea.

Place a tablet in the mouth or under the tongue if your pet seems unable to swallow it. Give a tablet every quarter of an hour. If necessary, the tablet may be crushed in a fold of paper and given with a dessertspoonful of boiled warm water. Frequent dosing for a couple of hours should stop the vomiting and the treatment may then be continued three times daily for a day or two until the condition has completely settled down.

Merc cor (Remedy 15): The animal is usually thirsty for large drinks of water which may be vomited back some hours later (in contrast to the previous symptoms, where arsenic is recommended). There is often diarrhoea associated with the vomiting and sometimes this is bloodstained.

Give one tablet every two hours on the first day and continue with a tablet four times daily for two or three days until the diarrhoea ceases.

Nux vomica (Remedy 17): For the more occasional vomiting associated with digestive upsets of one kind or another and when no marked increase in thirst is apparent. One tablet four hourly until relief.

WARTS

These are not usually serious but can be a nuisance and they sometimes get knocked and bleed or the animal begins to worry them and they have to be removed.

Treatment
The remedy Thuja has an effect on many warts but needs to be used under the guidance of a veterinary surgeon who uses homeopathy.
     Nitric acid is another remedy that can be used under supervision to treat warts.

WORMS

There are two main groups of worms that infect our pets – the roundworms and tapeworms or flat worms.

Roundworms
Roundworms are commonplace in young puppies and kittens. The roundworm that lives in the small intestine of dogs *(toxocara canis)* can be picked up by the puppy in the womb of the bitch, or through the milk, or by eating one of the many eggs that all parasites lay. The cat roundworm *(toxocara cati)* is not picked up by the kitten in the womb but may be in the mother's milk or be eaten as an egg or by the cat eating a small rodent that is carrying the worm itself. The third roundworm *(toxascaris leonina)* affects both dogs and cats. The worms may not be seen for months and in fact sometimes are only spotted because the

animal vomits and brings some up or passes
bout of diarrhoea.

Treatment
There are many safe and effective treatments for
available in the shops and from your veterinary s

Homoeopathic Remedy

Cina or *Santonin*: Before using these remedies, consult a
veterinary surgeon who uses homoeopathy.

Tapeworms

Tapeworms have very complicated life cycles involving passage
through an intermediate host or second animal (the flea or small
rodent or rabbit, depending on the particular tapeworm concerned)
before they can again infect their main host animal such as the
dog or cat.

The head of the tapeworm possesses strong suckers which
become embedded in the intestinal wall of the host and the
worm then produces segments and may grow to 20 or 30 inches
long (50-75 cm). The segments gradually ripen, become detached
from the end of the worm and fall out in the droppings or wriggle
out through the back passage. They may resemble the maggots
found in rotten meat and move rather like a caterpillar, or they
become dry and have the appearance of grains of rice. A dozen
or so segments may pass out daily and each contains many eggs.
These eggs then have to pass through the flea or other
intermediate host before reinfecting the main host.

The head of the tapeworm becomes lodged very firmly in the
intestinal wall and is difficult to expel, so tapeworm remedies
have to be powerful in action but harmless to the host animal.

Treatment

Granatum (Pomegranate)

The pomegranate has the power to expel tapeworms and can be
used homoeopathically.

WOUNDS

This word embraces numerous sorts of injury, from a simple small gash to an enormous tear or a deep, penetrating puncture. Whatever the cause or the size of the wound, the first action must be to clean it. Weak salt solution (about half a teaspoonful of ordinary household salt in approximately a pint [570ml] of warm water) is in my opinion just as good as any of the antiseptics or disinfectants for the cleaning of wounds. Once the wound is cleaned and, if possible, some hair cut away, the extent of it can be more easily assessed. If there is any question that it might need stitching, then the sooner this is done by your veterinary surgeon the better, before any natural but possibly unsatisfactory healing begins to take place.

Local Treatment
Calendula lotion has remarkable healing properties and should be applied locally two or three times daily to small wounds and abrasions.

Oral Treatment
To promote healing, and if there are signs of shock associated with a wound a few doses of arnica are very helpful.

Arnica (Remedy 3): A tablet given every two hours up to four doses and then three to four times daily for a few days.

Puncture wounds are often painful, as everybody knows who has been bitten by a cat or a dog. In such cases hypericum can be used, usually after a few doses of arnica have been given to control any shock and haemorrhage that may have occurred.

Hypericum (Remedy 14): One tablet every two to four hours or three to four times daily until the pain has obviously eased.

Footnote
It may not always be easy to know if your pet is suffering any pain but loss of appetite, restlessness or continual licking or

gnawing at a wound indicates discomfort or pain. It is possible to get Hypercal lotion or ointment (hypericum and calendula together) from your homoeopathic chemist which is excellent for treating wounds.

YAWNING

Some animals appear to yawn with pleasure or when they are tired and relaxing, others when they are bored and looking for mischief to get up to. Some yawn more often than others so, as with drinking habits, it is the pattern of yawning that may be significant.

Sudden repeated yawning usually means that your pet is out of sorts (as with car sickness, for instance) and remedial action should be taken.

Remedy

Chelidonium: A few doses of chelidonium (celandine) may ease the mild case due to overeating etc. which may have a temporary effect on the liver.

Nux vomica (Remedy 17): Nux vomica is useful in all digestive upsets. Give three or four doses at two to four hour intervals.

Persistent yawning, particularly if associated with other symptoms such as vomiting or diarrhoea, should be investigated.

2.
THE REMEDIES

THE VETERINARY PACK

I have selected twenty-four remedies that I have found useful in practice to treat most of the common conditions we might expect to find in our pets. These are intended as first-aid measures or 'before we call the vet' remedies that may be safely used while you decide if it is necessary to consult your veterinary surgeon. They are not intended to replace or be a substitute for the excellent veterinary services that are now available throughout the United States.

In an attempt to increase the interest of the reader in homoeopathy, I have deliberately given additional information when describing the remedies, including the origin and nature of the substance where possible and anecdotes about their homoeopathic use in man or animals.

At the end of the veterinary pack remedies I have listed other remedies that I have referred to in the text and given brief details about them and their particular action.

Remedy 1: Aconite *Shock – Burns – fever*

Aconitum napellus – Monk's-hood – Wolf's-bane
Family: Ranunculaceae

Aconite is a herbaceous perennial and a member of the buttercup family. It is a handsome but somehow sinister plant which contains aconitine, making it the most poisonous plant in Europe. The flowers are purplish-blue in colour and shaped like a monk's cowl. The plant flowers from June to August.

In homoeopathy it has been called the homoeopathic lancet because years ago it replaced the surgical instrument of that name which was used for 'blood-letting' in cases of acute fever. In those days, if blood-letting was not practised in acute conditions such as pneumonia or pleurisy, it was considered to be the equivalent to murder, for without blood-letting (or leeching) the patient must surely die.

Today we know that in fact blood-letting and the putting of blood-sucking leeches on the body in the mistaken belief that they sucked out the 'bad' blood containing the disease, did far more harm than good to a patient, who was probably already anaemic. Dr Hahnemann was one of the first doctors to appreciate this fact and campaigned for the use of his proven homoeopathic remedies in place of these barbaric practices.

Aconite was his chosen remedy to replace blood-letting in acute feverish conditions.

Uses: All cases of shock or fright from accidents or injuries and wounds, etc. Aconite is also indicated in the early, acute stages of fever such as in flu, pneumonia and septicaemia. Other possible uses include burns and scalds, snakebites and any haemorrhage (bleeding) accompanied by shock.

Dosage: One tablet every quarter of an hour if necessary, up to four or six doses, while deciding if further remedies or veterinary attention are required.

Remedy 2: Apis mel

Apis mellifica – The honey bee

Many of us enjoy eating honey and taken medicinally with hot lemon and whisky when we have a bad cold, it has a wonderfully warming effect – a cure in fact! Bees and their stings have been used for generations as a treatment in folk medicine.

I remember years ago seeing a television programme with an elderly lady who called herself 'the bloody old quack from Bromley', placing bees around a patient's knee and leaving the stings embedded around the joint for a while as a relief for arthritis. Homoeopathically, the whole bee – including the sting – is used to make the remedy apis mel.

Uses: Apis mel is used for painful bites and stings ('like treats like') and any condition where there is sudden swelling of the tissues (oedema). In humans, apis can be a marvellous remedy for sore throats when the throat and tonsils are swollen, fiery red with stinging pains and the sensation of a fishbone sticking in the throat. Before antibiotics, apis mel was used to good effect to treat the awful sore throat of diphtheria victims. Other uses include treatment for arthritis, abscesses, otitis (inflammation of the ear), acute conjunctivitis, incontinence and some cases of acute eczema. There is no increased thirst and the animal that one might treat with apis will be seeking the cold stone, concrete or lino floor to lie upon; it will not be wanting to sit by the fire or the radiator.

Dosage: For acute cases such as stings or insect bites, one tablet every hour up to four tablets, then one three or four times daily for a day or two until relief in less acute conditions.

Summary of Apis Mel in Verse

> Honey – bee – Apis – its virtues we sing
> For all manner of pains that burn and sting,
> With bad aggravations from all kinds of heat,
> With puffings and swellings and tension: repeat,
> Till you've got it by heart, that the Bee is the thing,
> For all manner of pains that burn and sting.

Remedy 3: Arnica   *Shock – Bruising*

Arnica montana – Leopard's bane – Mountain tobacco
Family: Compositae – the daisy family

Arnica is a perennial plant with bright yellow flowers and at the base of each stem a rosette of oval leaves pressed to the ground surface. It flowers in July and August and it grows in the mountain regions and has been used as an infusion for topical application from very early times. In Switzerland, apparently, arnica is popular among skiers for treating knocks, sprains and bruises of all kinds. In fact, arnica is one of the most valued and useful of our homoeopathic remedies.

Uses: Arnica is indicated before and after dental work, such as extractions and, in fact, before and after any operation or in any instance when there is shock, haemorrhage or bruising. Arnica is known affectionately as the *panacea lapsorum*, a sort of cure for all ills, and rightly so. If other remedies are not to hand, arnica could be used for sores of any kind, abscesses (boils), dislocations, fractures and obvious tooth discomfort. It is indicated in all cases of strain and over-exercise (after a day's shooting or a sudden, extra-long walk causing stiffness) and also for wasp stings. Any bruising after parturition (giving birth) will soon respond to a few doses of arnica.

Other uses include any accident, anaemia, anal gland problems, aural haematoma and other haemorrhages (e.g. nosebleeds),

bites, bruises of all kinds, snakebites, frights, sh
paraplegia (paralysis of the hind limbs).

I think it can be safely said that for almost any coi ..ttion
arnica will certainly do no harm and in many instances is most
beneficial. It is a short-acting remedy and may need to be
repeated frequently, but its action is rapid.

Dosage: One tablet every two hours up to four or six doses,
followed by one four times daily for a few days until relief is
apparent.

Remedy 4: Arsenic

Arsenicum album – White arsenic – Arsenic trioxide

Arsenic trioxide, to give it its correct chemical name, occurs as a
heavy white powder. The poison arsenic is so widely known that
almost everybody at some time must have read a novel or story
in which the victim was poisoned with it. When arsenic trioxide
is mixed with sugar it is difficult to distinguish and, once eaten,
causes terrible burning pains with severe attacks of vomiting
and diarrhoea. Arsenic, like arnica and rhus tox, is one of our
most wide-ranging and versatile homoeopathic remedies. It has
a deep-seated activity on every organ and part of the body and is
able to increase 'the feeling of well-being' rather like taking a
drink does for many people. This helps to make the patient,
human or animal, feel better and aids recovery in this way.

Uses: Arsenic is absolutely symptomatic in the treatment of
acute vomiting and diarrhoea and should be given as soon as
possible after the condition starts.

It is also useful for acute conjunctivitis, sneezing, fever,
septicaemia, all forms of enteritis (parvovirus infection), loss of
appetite, chronic metritis and skin conditions such as chronic
eczema and dandruff (scurf).

Dosage: In acute cases give one tablet every quarter to half an hour, up to six or eight doses if necessary. This may be followed by giving one tablet four times daily for two or three days, which should be sufficient in most instances. In skin conditions a course of three days' treatment may be repeated after an interval of one to two weeks if it appears to be giving relief.

Remedy 5: Bryonia

Bryonia alba – White bryony – Wild hops
Family: Cucurbitaceae – The pumpkin family

Bryony is a common perennial. It has a massive, twisted white root which, it is said, has been sold by rogues in the past as a substitute for mandrake roots, reputed from biblical times to be an aphrodisiac. It is, in fact, a poisonous plant and flowers from May to September with greenish-yellow flowers, followed by red berries.

Uses: One very strong symptom that indicates the use of bryonia is that whatever the condition, it becomes worse with movement. Bryonia may be used to treat arthritis, rheumatism (only when both are worse for moving), chest infections, nosebleeds and mastitis. There is a dryness inside the mouth and the animal will appear thirsty. There may be a dry, harsh cough, as in 'kennel cough', which always becomes worse with movement. Bryonia indicates very well the principle of homoeopathy that the symptoms must exactly fit the choice of remedy. I have had some very encouraging results with bryonia, but have also been equally disappointed when I have obviously decided to use it for the wrong reasons.

Dosage: One tablet four times daily for several days. The conditions that respond to bryonia usually take some time to develop and correspondingly the response to the remedy may take some days to show.

Remedy 6: Cantharis

Lytta vesicatoria – Spanish fly
Family: Meloidae – oil beetles

cystitis

This insect, which is green in colour and looks more like a winged beetle than a fly, occurs in Europe (mainly central and southern) and Siberia. It feeds on the leaves of ash, lilac, privet and other plants and lays its eggs near the nests of solitary bees. The larvae that hatch from the eggs make their way into the bee's nest and develop there (metamorphosis) into the Spanish fly which emerges mostly in June and July. The fly itself contains a quantity of the toxic chemical substance cantharidin, which was used as a medicine by doctors in ancient times and right up to the Renaissance. It was also used as a poison.

Many colourful stories of the effectiveness of Spanish fly as an aphrodisiac (sexual stimulant) have been told and retold by countless schoolboys over the years and no doubt much exaggerated in the telling. It is no exaggeration, however, to say that cantharides is an extremely powerful irritant and as it is passed out in the urine, far from causing sexual arousement, is much more likely to induce severe, raw, burning pains, driving the taker almost to the point of frenzy.

Fortunately, homoeopathically, all the harmful and distressing powers of this substance are removed and we are left with a soothing and reliable remedy for many sorts of burning pain.

Uses: Acute and chronic cystitis, some kinds of nephritis (kidney problems), gnat bites, stings, scalds and any other burning or blistery sores including some acute forms of eczema.

Dosage: One tablet every hour up to four or six tablets, then one four times daily until relief.

Remedy 7: Carbo veg

Carbo vegetabilis – Vegetable charcoal

In early times it was thought that wood charcoal was inert and of little use. Later it was discovered that it could remove bad odours and smells from the breath and the bowels (up or down!). Dr Hahnemann took this apparently inactive substance and potentized it to produce a valuable remedy.

Uses: Flatulence (wind) of all sorts, constipation accompanied by wind, collapse and the shock associated with it. It may also be of use in treating chronic nosebleeding with sneezing.

Dosage: In cases of collapse a tablet can be placed under the tongue or crushed between a fold of clean paper and the powder put inside the lips or poured onto the tongue. This can be repeated every five to fifteen minutes if necessary, while help is being summoned.

For the treatment of flatulence the tablet may be given on every occasion when there is evidence of wind, possibly an hour before a meal in the animal that constantly has this offensive and antisocial condition.

Footnote
Carbo veg is known to many homoeopathic physicians as the 'corpse reviver', because it has apparently done just that on occasions when a patient has collapsed and appeared to be on the point of death.

Remedy 8: Chamomilla

Painst mucus mebranes

Matricaria chamomilla – Wild camomile – Scented mayweed
Family: Compositae – The daisy family

The word chamomilla comes from the Greek words meaning

'apples on the ground'. This is because when the petals have gone, the flower-heads resemble tiny pineapples to look at and also have the scent of pineapple or apples. In fact, scented mayweed was a well-known folklore remedy to our ancestors who made camomile tea from infusing the dried flower-heads in boiling water and used it as a cure for indigestion and insomnia. Camomile is widespread and found in gardens, building sites, hedgerows, waste-ground and even cultivated fields. The daisy-like flowers can be seen from May to September.

Uses: All types of pain, particularly toothache, earache, any sign of pain at teething (more in babies than puppies, kittens, etc.) and in painful conditions such as mastitis.

Dosage: Frequent doses, every five to fifteen minutes, may be given if needed, or at one to two hourly intervals for less acute cases until relief is apparent.

Remedy 9: Cocculus

Cocculus indicus – Indian cockle seed
Family: Menispermaceae

Dr Edward Hamilton, in his *Flora Homoeopathica* published in 1852, writes: 'The importation of the drug *(cocculus indicus)* into this country is considerably less in quantity than formerly, and is seldom used unless it is for the illicit adulteration of beer and porter in low public houses!' Apparently it has an inebriating quality which stimulates added strength to the liquor. It also prevents the secondary fermentation of beer, and bursting of the bottles in warm climates. (What about that, home-brew experts?)

The plant *anamirta cocculus* which contains the seed *cocculus indicus* is a strong, climbing plant with small, yellow flowers and it grows in the Indian archipelago and on the coast of Malabar (the south-west coast of India). The berry from which the seed is derived resembles the berry of the bay tree and contains the powerful poison picrotoxin. In ancient times this poison was used to stupefy fish which made them easier to catch.

Uses: The older books talk about cocculus being used as a homoeopathic treatment for sickness from 'riding in a carriage', an expression which I like very much.

In modern times this means the 'motion sickness' of any form of travel by car, boat or air (it might even help astronauts!). It can also be used to treat some forms of epilepsy (fits).

Dosage: Give one tablet thirty to forty minutes before the start of the journey.

For fits one tablet four hourly may help to control this distressing condition.

Remedy 10: Colocynth

Colocynthis – Citrullus colocynthis – known variously as Bitter apple, bitter or squirting cucumber.
Family: Cucurbitaceae – The pumpkin family

This variety of the pumpkin family is a gourd and grows naturally in Turkey. Squirting cucumbers were certainly plants of ancient cultivation but were not grown in Britain until the sixteenth century when they are mentioned in a book called *Turner's Herball* of 1568. The squirting cucumber is an interesting plant, being so called because when it is ripe the slightest touch will cause the small, black seeds to be discharged and propelled anything from six to fifteen feet (2-5m).

Uses: Colocynth is a fine pain remedy for acute pains in the abdomen. The horse with severe colic immediately comes to mind, because its characteristic symptoms of looking round at the side, kicking at the belly and getting up and down (i.e., extreme restlessness) and, if in agony, rolling from side to side are symptomatic of the colocynth pain. The human patient with

colic that will benefit from colocynth has the sort c
pain that bends him double. Colic may be seen
domestic pets from time to time, usually from eating s
out of the ordinary, but the symptoms may not be q.e so
dramatic as those outlined above for the horse.

Dosage: One tablet every quarter of an hour until relief.

N.B. Seek veterinary attention immediately if acute colic is
suspected in any animal.

Remedy 11: Euphrasia

Euphrasia officinalis – Eyebright
Family: Scrophulariaceae – The figwort family

How interesting that this little plant called 'Eyebright' by our
ancestors should have been used successfully for hundreds of
years for treating eye conditions. Euphrasia is a common plant
in grassland and pastures and is found throughout Europe. It is
an annual and it flowers from June to September. The two-
lipped flower has a smaller upper petal and a larger lower one,
both being snow-white in colour but streaked with purple and
having a yellow blotch near the middle.

Uses: Local application as an eyewash or in an eyebath. One drop
of the mother tincture in an eye-bath or eggcupful of boiled
warm water makes an excellent solution for bathing the eyes.
The eyes may be bathed once or twice daily and this treatment
helps to relieve acute and chronic conjunctivitis and watering
eyes (from allergies etc.).

Note: A mother tincture is the concentrated form of the plant or
substance (e.g. mercury, sulphur, etc.) prepared by extraction
and filtration in a mixture of pure alcohol and pure water.

Internal Use: Euphrasia tablets may be useful to treat some allergies, catarrh, acute and chronic conjunctivitis and cataract.

Dosage: One tablet every two hours up to four doses, followed by one three or four times daily until relief.

Remedy 12: Gelsemium *flu—fever + fear*

Gelsemium sempervirens – Yellow jasmine
Family: Loganiaceae – The buddleia group of plants that attract the butterflies

This is a climbing plant that grows in the southern states of America and was discovered as a homoeopathic remedy by an American, Dr E. M. Hale, who introduced a number of useful remedies and produced a book about them.

Gelsemium is a wonderful 'flu' remedy for humans and among its other properties it is able to dispel the bad effects of anticipation such as diarrhoea before exams or going to the dentist etc. The remedy is prepared from the fresh root and contains two alkaloids, one of which – gelseminine – acts like strychnine.

Uses: For animals we can use gelsemium for fever, sneezing, flu (especially cat flu) and for fear. Gelsemium is the remedy for 'shaking with fright'.

Dosage: For flu, fever, etc., one tablet every two hours on the first day, then one four times daily until relief. For fear and fright, give one tablet every hour up to four doses if necessary.

Remedy 13: Hepar sulph

Hepar sulphuris – Calcium sulphide

This is one of the remedies developed by Dr Hahnemann and *Hepar sulphuris calcareum* is still prepared according to his directions from a mixture of equal parts of finely powdered oyster shells and pure flowers of sulphur kept at white heat for ten minutes.

Uses: It is when there is a tendency to suppuration or the production of pus in part of the body that hepar sulph is so useful; for example, abscesses of all kinds, anal gland infections, middle ear disease and infected otitis, infected gums (gingivitis), chronic tonsillitis, dermatitis and mastitis, etc.

Dosage: One tablet every two hours up to four doses, then one tablet three times daily for three to four days.

Remedy 14: Hypericum

Hypericum perforatum – St John's wort
Family: Hypericaceae

St John's wort has been known since the first century AD and in the Middle Ages when superstitions were widely believed it was thought to have the power to cast out demons. In those early days, if Christian prayers failed to rid a woman of a devil she was thought to possess she would place the leaves of St John's wort on her bosom and about her home to send the demon on its way. Certainly a lotion made from the plant can be used to dress wounds and is soothing for burns. The flowers are golden yellow and are found growing wild just about everywhere from June to September.

Uses: Hypericum is a remedy that eases pain particularly after bites and other painful blows and wounds. It may also be helpful in cases of paralysis such as paraplegia.

Dosage: One tablet every two to four hours or three or four tablets daily until the pain has obviously lessened.

Footnote: Pain is sometimes difficult to appreciate in an animal unless it cries out and the exact place which is painful may not be obvious. The signs of pain are usually restlessness, panting or sweating, loss of appetite and continual licking, rubbing or sometimes scratching of the painful part. In more severe cases when pain is involved, there may be vomiting and diarrhoea and the animal may throw itself about and writhe around on the ground (e.g. with colic).

Remedy 15: Merc cor

Mercurius corrosivus – Corrosive sublimate Hg Cl$_2$

The corrosive sublimate of mercury (see also *Merc Sol*, Remedy 16) is so called because it is just that – a powerful substance that corrodes and irritates what it comes in contact with. Internally, poisoning with mercury causes violent gastroenteritis and on the 'like for like' basis this is what we use it for homoeopathically – to treat persistent and sometimes haemorrhagic diarrhoea often accompanied by vomiting with acute abdominal pain. There is usually great thirst and the water is vomited back later, in contrast to the arsenic D and V (diarrhoea and vomiting) when the water is thrown up again almost immediately. Mercury has been used in medicine for some hundreds of years and the signs and symptoms of over-dosage were all too well known to physicians at one time. Chronic mercury poisoning closely follows the pattern of the symptoms and signs seen in progressive cases of syphilis (venereal disease) and it was therefore widely used by the earlier homoeopaths to treat this condition.

Uses: Acute enteritis and dysentery (bloody diarrhoea with much straining), Parvovirus infection (in conjunction with fluid and other conventional therapy), middle ear infections and sometimes for incontinence.

Dosage: One tablet two hourly up to four doses, then one three times daily for two to three days, should be sufficient in many cases.

Remedy 16: Merc sol

Mercurius solubilis – Quicksilver

We all know the heavy, silver-coloured, liqu
out of the thermometer when we drop it a
critical moment. Metals (like most other thing
get hot and this is how the thermometer work   ne thin
column of mercury sliding up the scale as it gets warm from the
body temperature.

Mercury makes a fine homoeopathic remedy and Dr
Hahnemann himself developed the use of the black oxide of
mercury, which we know as merc sol.

Uses: It has a more gentle but much wider range of activity than
merc cor. Merc sol is indicated in cases of acute wet eczema,
including eczema of the ear flap, acute and chronic nephritis,
chronic diarhoea and swollen, red gums with offensive breath.

Dosage: One tablet every two hours on the first day, followed by
one four times daily for five to ten days, according to the
condition being treated.

Remedy 17: Nux vomica

Strychnos nux vomica – Poison-nut
Family: Locaniaceae – The buddlia family

The tree from which the nux vomica seeds come is of considerable
size with grey, knobbly bark. It grows in Vietnam and Indonesia
and the fruit, about the size of a large apple, is bright orange in
colour when ripe and this attracts birds who eat it readily. In this
way the seeds are distributed and each piece of fruit contains
two to five seeds. The seeds contain two very poisonous
alkaloids – strychnine and brucine, but because the nut is so
bitter to the taste it is an uncommon poison. It has been used as a

_cinal substance since early times and some may remember the tonic 'Eastern Syrup' which contained minute traces of strychnine and was said to be a cure for boils. The poison strychnine in material doses causes the most violent muscular spasms and convulsions resulting in death, with the body becoming completely rigid. It used to be one of the methods employed to destroy animals but fortunately nowadays, has been superseded by giving overdoses of the anaesthetic pentobarbitone (Nembutal).

Uses: In humans this is the remedy for overindulgence – too much to eat and too much to drink – in fact, a good 'hangover' remedy. In animals it may be used for chronic forms of colic with constipation and flatulence, bad breath, loss of appetite and digestive upsets, hiccups, hepatitis and jaundice. It is also helpful in cases of 'slipped disc'.

Dosage: One tablet every four hours until relief. A tablet may be given every two hours up to four doses in more urgent cases, but on the whole this is a remedy that is most helpful in chronic conditions.

Remedy 18: Pulsatilla *pining shy – mucous membrane*

Pulsatilla nigricans – Meadow anemone, the pasque-flower or windflower
Family: Ranunculaceae – The buttercup family

This rather delicate-looking but pretty, violet-purple flower is found among grasses on dry, chalky, windy slopes throughout Britain and in most of Europe. It is a perennial plant and flowers twice a year in May and again in August or September. In homoeopathy the remedy is prepared from the juice of the whole plant.

Uses: Homoeopathic physicians widely employ pulsatilla to

treat rather depressed, sad people with a variety of ailments and it seems to suit rather passive, mild dispositions. In animals we can carry forward this concept to a certain extent too and treat the condition of 'pining' for the owner who is absent.

Pulsatilla is also useful in treating cases of chronic catarrh, false pregnancy and agalactia (shortage of milk) in the bitch. A few doses of pulsatilla at parturition (giving birth) can be most beneficial. It may also be helpful in toothache, incontinence, mastitis and some liver complaints, particularly in conditions where there seems to be an improvement when the animal is outside rather than in a warm place.

Dosage: One tablet every four hours until relief. Treatment may be continued for a few days if it appears to be beneficial and in parturition cases it may be given every thirty to forty minutes until the process is complete.

Remedy 19: Rhus tox

Rhus toxicondendron – Poison Ivy or Poison Oak
Family: Anacardiaceae – The ivy family

This is one of my favourite remedies because it is the one that convinced me that homoeopathy really works for the simple reason that it worked on me! I have been a 'bad back' sufferer for more than fifteen years, but after attending my first course in homoeopathic medicine at the Royal Homoeopathic Hospital in London, I decided to take rhus tox myself. It has worked wonders and my back is now better than it has been for years.

The plant grows freely in the United States of America and Canada. The stems trail along the ground like our own ivy and climb when they find the support of a wall or a tree, etc. The flowers appear in June and July. The homoeopathic remedy is prepared from a tincture of fresh leaves gathered in May during the evening, because the sunlight not only turns the milky-white juice black but renders it inactive. Rhus tox has many actions, but two of the principal ones are the treatment of rheumatic-type pains and its effect on the skin. Touching or even brushing against the leaves of the plant will cause acute urticaria (nettle-rash), with intense irritation and the formation of blisters.

Uses: The sorts of arthritis, rheumatism and muscular disorders that respond well to rhus tox are those that are at their worst after periods of rest, but the pain and stiffness ease a little once movement has commenced. It may also be used to treat fevers, flu accompanied by a bad cough, septicaemia, sprains and strains and various skin conditions such as some acute and chronic forms of eczema.

Dosage: In acute disorders one tablet every two hours up to four or six doses on the first day, followed by one four times a day for a few days if necessary until relief.

Footnote: My brother once suffered from an attack of shingles and the best the doctor could offer was applications of spirit (shaving lotion) to the affected area and aspirins for the persistent headache. After several days of considerable discomfort I heard of his illness and immediately sent a course of rhus tox selected on the symptoms he described. He began to improve within a few hours of taking the first tablet and now goes round telling everybody that his shingles was cured by the vet and not the doctor. It is interesting to add that it was the spontaneous cure of herpetic lesions (like those of shingles) in a young man who accidentally rubbed against a poison-ivy plant that first gave physicians the idea that it could be used medicinally. This was over two hundred years ago and rhus had probably been employed by herbalists and monks long before this.

Remedy 20: Scutellaria

Scutellaria lateriflora – Skullcap or mad-dog
Family: Labiatae – The mint family

Skullcap is so called because of the distinctive shape of the flower, which is like a two-lipped tube with a broad pouch-like scale at the back, and this distinguishes it from the rest of the mint family. Two varieties occur naturally in the United Kingdom and the skullcap plant grows from about six to twenty inches (15-50cm) in height. The blue flowers appear from June to September and are found in wet places such as water-meadows and by streams. The skullcap plant contains a volatile oil called scutellarin which has been known for many years to be a treatment for nervous disorders. It is not surprising, therefore, that homoeopathically it is also an excellent 'nerve' remedy and could almost be described as the homoeopathic tranquillizer.

Uses: Nervous conditions of all sorts, apprehension, strange behaviour patterns, chorea, fits (epilepsy) and juvenile delinquent puppies!

Dosage: One tablet twice daily for up to a week if necessary. After a few doses improvement may be evident and in such cases cease treatment for a while and assess results. Repeat treatment only if required.

Remedy 21: Silica

Silica – Silicon dioxide – Pure flint, sand

What can one say about something like sand except that it is found everywhere and is very hard and gritty when you are on the beach and get it in your mouth?

In ordinary medicine silica as a remedy is more or less unknown, being considered inert, but when prepared for

it passes into a colloidal state which has a
on the animal's body. Silica is found in the
ny plants and occurs in minute amounts in the
animal body including the dental enamel. Too
much inhaled as a dust over a long period, as we know can
cause the harmful, sometimes fatal, disease silicosis. Mineral
waters, on the other hand, contain traces of silica which can be
beneficial to the body.

Uses: It is an excellent remedy for chronic conditions and where
there is infection and sepsis (with pus formation). It follows well
after treatment with hepar sulph in the acute phase (Remedy
13).

The chronic conditions that come to mind where silica may
well help or follow ordinary treatment are anal gland infection,
chronic conjunctivitis, corneal ulcer, recurrent sore throat,
middle ear disease, broken nails, foreign bodies such as grass
seeds and mastitis, etc.

Dosage: One tablet given three times daily for ten days. It may
be necessary to persist with one tablet, say, twice daily for a long
time in really chronic conditions such as broken nails, corneal
ulcer and cataract.

Remedy 22: Sulphur

Sulphur sublimatum – Flowers of sulphur

The element sulphur can be obtained by sublimation of native
sulphur or as a by-product of refining crude petroleum. At one
time a lump of yellow sulphur was commonplace in the dog's
water bowl, deemed to be a conditioner particularly of the skin.
Sulphur is only very slightly soluble in water so what good it did,
if any, is questionable. Sulphur is, however, one of the oldest
remedies in medicine and has been widely used in skin
applications and also as a purgative.

Once prepared for homoeopathic use it becomes a very potent remedy; it was much used by Dr Hahnemann and is still very popular with homoeopaths today.

Sulphur, which is an invariable constituent of albumen (an essential body protein), is found in nearly all the different tissues of the body but particularly in the epithelial tissues (the tissues related to skin). Sulphur, therefore, has a profound action in the treatment of many skin conditions and is of special use in the treatment of chronic diseases.

Uses: Skin conditions, acute dry eczema, chronic dermatitis, puritus, dandruff, mange, conjunctivitis, chronic diarrhoea, chronic fever, pneumonia, incontinence and chronic rheumatism. In fact, a very wide variety of diseases and conditions may well respond to treatment with sulphur if it is selected for the right reasons.

Dosage: Sulphur often produces its best results when used sparingly. Give one tablet twice daily for two to five days and then wait a week or two to assess results.

Footnote: Sulphur is a remedy that may well need the skill of a homoeopath to obtain the best results from its use.

Remedy 23: Symphytum

Symphytum officinale – common comfrey – 'Boneset'
Family: Boraginaceae – The forget-me-not family

Common comfrey is widespread throughout Europe and Northern Asia and grows in damp places. The flowering season is May to July and the flowers may be cream, white, purple or pink, but only one colour appears on each plant. In medieval times the comfrey root was grated into a sludge and packed round fractures where it soon became hard rather like plaster of Paris is used today. Hence the folklore names 'boneset' and 'knitbone'. Incidentally, the word 'officinal' means a drug sold in an apothecary's (chemist's) shop.

Uses: The principal use of comfrey is in the treatment of fractures and especially those that fail to unite readily. It may also be useful in the treatment of sprains and strains and has a special place in the relief of pain from injuries to the eye, from a blow or a knock.

Dosage: After a fracture has been treated by whatever means by your veterinary surgeon, I would recommend a course of treatment with comfrey. Give one tablet three times daily for ten to fourteen days.

For eye injuries give a tablet every two hours up to four doses and then one four times daily for two to three days.

Remedy 24: Urtica

Urtica urens – The small nettle
Family: Urticaceae – The stinging-nettle family

It is difficult to imagine that the common stinging nettle which is found in almost every hedgerow, farmyard, field and a good many gardens, too, can be a useful remedy. The small nettle, which seldom grows to a foot in height, is found throughout Europe but is slightly less common than the ordinary stinging nettle and flowers from May to October. Years ago nettle tea was used as an infusion (the dry leaves soaked in hot water) and taken internally for fevers. It was also used externally as a tincture in lotions or compresses to treat burns and scalds. Throughout the centuries man can be said to have had a real 'love-hate relationship' with the lowly nettle; on the one hand cursing it for its stinging properties and its widespread and persistent distribution, yet at the same time employing it as a valuable medicine. It is even said that medieval monks beat their bare backs with nettles as a means of torture.

Dosage: One tablet every fifteen minutes up to four doses, then one every two to three hours for up to twelve hours, by which time the acute condition should have resolved.

Footnote: If anybody would like to put the truth of homoeopathy (i.e., that 'like cures like') crudely to the test it can be done with nettles. Handle a few strong fresh nettles with bare hands and you will readily find that they *do* produce a rash.

Treatment with nettle-tea or a few doses of nettle tincture in water or urtica tablets (from your vet pack) will give speedy relief.

Other useful remedies that could be kept with the Veterinary Pack:

Euphrasia Eye Drops
Mother tincture – for directions regarding use see *Eye Conditions – Acute Conjunctivitis.*

Burn Ointment
A burn ointment is available from homoeopathic chemists and is stocked in jars or tubes. The ointment contains hypericum to relieve the pain and urtica to ease the irritation and soothe the stinging. This should be applied frequently to burns, scalds and sores of all kinds.

Hypericum/Calendula Ointment
Hypericum/calendula ointment is also soothing and applied four or five times daily, could be used as an alternative to the burn ointment for treating wounds.

Chelidonium majus – Common celandine. For liver conditions (see hepatitis), jaundice, yawning.

Cina – Worm seed. For roundworms.

ADDITIONAL REMEDIES MENTIONED IN THE BOOK AND THEIR USES

I had not appreciated as I was writing this book that I had referred to quite so many other remedies (another twenty-four) in addition to the twenty-four in the veterinary pack. However, it does help to demonstrate the fact that it is an important principle of homoeopathy to select exactly the right remedy to suit the symptom picture if a good response is to be achieved.

Allium cepa – The onion. Persistent tears and cat flu.

Baryta carb – Barium carbonate. 'The old age remedy' for senility.

Borax – Sodium borate. Colourless crystals or a white powder used as a weak antiseptic in a mouthwash or an eye lotion. Homoeopathically for sudden loud frightening noises, e.g. fireworks.

Caulophyllum – Blue cohosh or squaw root. So called because North American Indian women chewed the root at the time the birth of a baby was imminent and they seldom had any obstetrical problems. Caullophyllum could easily have been one of the remedies in the vet pack and I strongly commend it to anybody who is in the business of breeding. One tablet of potency twelve or thirty given daily for three to four weeks before the event can ease the birth process.

Causticum – Potassium hydroxide. One of Dr Hahnemann's original remedies, used for chorea, paraplegia and warts.

Uses: Urticaria (nettle-rash) and other allergic conditions of the skin with extreme redness and irritation, e.g. acute allergic eczema. It is also used to treat agalactia (lack of milk secretion).

Conium maculatum – Poison hemlock. For arthritis, progressive weakness of hind limbs and paraplegia.

Croton tiglium – Croton oil seeds. For chronic long-standing diarrhoea, intense skin irritation, almost too tender to scratch.

Granatum – Pomegranate – Grenadine. The juice of the pomegranate is an ingredient of some cocktails. Homoeopathically it is a remedy for tapeworms.

Graphites – Black lead. For ear infections, chronic wet, sticky eczema.

Hamamelis virginica – Witch hazel. For bruising, bleeding (from nose etc.), wounds, chronic effects of injuries.

Ignatia – St Ignatius bean. For pining, away from the owner.

Kali bich – Potassium bichromate. For chronic catarrhal conditions.

Phytolacca – Poke root. For mastitis, some rheumatic conditions.

Psorinum – The scabies vesicle (the cause of mange). This was Dr Hahnemann's first 'nosode', a disease product for the cure of disease (rather like vaccination today). This was a continuation of his theory 'like cures like'. Also for certain skin conditions under the guidance of a homoeopath.

Quinine – Cinchona bark – China officinalis. It was quinine that originally revealed the art of homoeopathy to Dr Hahnemann. He took minute doses of quinine and was able to reproduce almost exactly the symptoms of malaria. Also for anaemia, haemorrhages.

Ruta – Rue bitterwort. An ancient herb, supposed to be valuable against the influence of witches. For injuries to periosteum (the outer layer or 'skin' of bones), sprains and strains.

Sabina – Savine, a conifer. For metritis.

Santonin – The flower-heads of worm seed, Cina, a remedy for roundworms.

Sepia – The ink of the cuttlefish. What a strange substance to think of making into a homoeopathic remedy! A much-favoured remedy with homoeopathic physicians mainly for various female problems, metritis (inflammation of the womb), false pregnancy in the bitch.

Spongia – Roasted turkey sponge. I do not know who first thought of roasting turkey sponge and making a remedy of it. It was the first homoeopathic remedy that I came across many years ago when working in a south-east London practice. The clients frequently returned for bottles of 'pink heart cough' medicine. For the dry, harsh bouts of coughing seen in older and often overweight dogs and occasionally cats.

Tellurium – The metal. For itching skin conditions, ringworm.

Thuja – Arbor vitae – the tree of life, also known as white cedar, a conifer. Thuja acts on the skin and is used for treating warts; it may also be useful if there are ill-effects following vaccination.

EIGHT DESERT ISLAND REMEDIES
OR THE MINI-PACK

If I was to be wrecked on a desert island with my family and pets I would like to think I had at least the following eight remedies with me, as well as the eight gramophone records and the inexhaustible supply of needles!

Arnica, arsenic, cantharis, colocynth, hepar sulph, merc sol, rhus tox, sulphur.

As we bumped ashore there would bound to be shock and some bruising so we would all take a few doses of arnica to settle us down. The strange change of diet might give us all, even the dogs, some vomiting and diarrhoea so the arsenic would come in very handy. A change of water often upsets people and animals causing colic pains, so we would be glad of the colocynth, too. There would probably be all sorts of insects and stinging plants on the island so we should need the cantharis and the merc sol would be useful, too, if patches of wet eczema followed or we got a chill in the kidneys from the exposure. The dog might tread on a thorn, the cat get an abscess or one of the children tonsillitis so we could reach for the hepar sulph. After building the hut or after the dogs have chased about the island all day with their new-found freedom we might be very stiff – rhus tox would be the answer here. It might be quite difficult to keep ourselves really clean, or if any of us developed skin lesions such as dry eczema or dermatitis or went down with a fever or our elderly cats suffered chronic rheumatism, sulphur would bring relief.

3.
HOMOEOPATHY
FOR THOSE IN A HURRY

This is a copy of the sheet that I hand out in the surgery when I dispense homoeopathic remedies for animals. I include it here because it is a summary of the origins of homoeopathy, its aims and the storage and use of the various remedies. For these reasons I hope it will be useful as a short guide to the whole subject of this book.

Homoeopathy

Homoeopathy is a natural healing process and the remedies act to stimulate the body's own defence mechanisms to assist the patient (human and animal) to regain normal health. The word homoeopathy is derived from two Greek words, 'homoios' meaning 'like' and 'pathos' meaning 'suffering' or, in this context, illness or disease. Homoeopathy is therefore the medical (or veterinary) practice of treating like with like. This principle was well known to Hippocrates, the architect of medicine, and therefore dates back to the time of the ancient Greeks. However, it was a German physician in the eighteenth century (1796), Dr Samuel Hahnemann, who confirmed the remarkable discovery that what a drug could cause it could also cure. Dr Hahnemann was convinced that the existing medical practices of his day very often did more harm than good (e.g. blood-letting, leeches and material doses of such substances as arsenic and phosphorus). He therefore set out to look for an alternative which would be safe, gentle and effective.

Homoeopathy does not claim to take the place of conventional medicine, but rather to be used alongside ordinary medicine (known as allopathy) where it has been shown that it can help. Homoeopathy is also useful in chronic conditions which have not responded to the usual lines of treatment. During the last fifty years conventional medicine has expanded tremendously with many marvellous results and the manufacture and production of medicines is a multi-million dollar industry. Unfortunately, in some cases, the more powerful the drug the more drastic the side-effects and in the end the conditions caused by the side-effects are worse than the original ailment or disease. Homoeo-pathy, on the other hand, is harmless and the work of Dr Hahnemann can be summarized as follows:

1. A substance which when taken in large doses will produce symptoms of disease, for example arsenic, which causes vomiting and diarrhoea, can be used in homoeopathic potency to treat similar symptoms brought on by food poisoning or infection.

2. The extreme dilution of the remedies increases the curative properties and all the poisonous or undesirable effects are lost.

3. In human beings and to some extent with animals, the homoeopathic medicines are prescribed by the study of the whole person or animal (temperament etc.) rather than treating the specific disease or condition concerned.

Taking Homoeopathic Medicines

1. Keep the remedy in the container supplied.

2. Store away from strong light, great heat and from exposure to strong odours (moth-balls etc.).

3. The medicines are usually supplied as tablets or individual veterinary doses (powders).

4. Each dose should be given at least half an hour before or after

a meal. If the animal will only take the dose with foo
tablet in a small morsel of bread or some favourite

Dogs: The tablets are slightly sweet and for this reason the dog
will often chew them or lick them off your clean hand.
Alternatively, put them in the mouth or crush them to a powder
in a fold of clean paper and tip them onto the tongue.

Cats: Give as for dogs, or if necessary, powder the tablets and
mix them with a very small quantity of butter and place in the
cat's mouth.

Frequency of Dosage

1. Urgent, acute attacks – give one tablet every fifteen minutes
   up to four doses, then one tablet every two hours for up to
   another four doses.

2. Less urgent conditions – give one tablet three times daily for
   two to three days as directed.

3. Long-standing or chronic conditions – one tablet three times
   daily for four to seven days and repeat as directed.

4. Veterinary doses (individual powders) should be given as
   instructed.

Response to Treatment in Acute Cases

1. An improvement will sometimes be noticed within a few
   hours of the commencement of treatment. In more long-
   standing conditions the benefit may not be seen until a few
   days after the completion of the course of treatment.

2. Occasionally an 'aggravation' or transient worsening of the
   condition may occur at the commencement of treatment.
   This is not a cause for worry, but cease treatment for twenty-
   four hours and then continue as before, or consult the
   veterinary surgeon in charge of the case if you are at all
   worried.

3. Homoeopathy is no different from allopathy (conventional
    medicine) in that it does not always produce relief or a cure
    but it is absolutely certain that it is harmless.

CONCLUSION

If you have done what I often do, picked up a book and opened it at the back, then I can assure you that it makes little difference in this instance. I hope this is a book that people will feel able to dip into from time to time and find the information they are looking for. You can just as easily read on from here going gently through the *Potted Homoeopathy* or *Summary* section, followed by the *Eight Desert Island Remedies* and reach the two main sections in this way.

I hope that I have been able to interest the reader in the idea of homoeopathy not only for the household pet but also very much for the whole family, so that everybody may benefit from this wide-ranging but gentle form of healing. It was a doctor with his own great enthusiasm for homoeopathy who first got me interested in the subject and it is my wish to return that initiative and to get other people fascinated in this alternative form of medicine, not only for their pets but for themselves, too.

I would like to finish by mentioning a passage written by Dr Hahnemann himself almost two hundred years ago, soon after he qualified as a doctor. The article was entitled: 'Directions for Curing Old Sores and Indolent Ulcers'. In this article he made a scathing attack on the accepted methods of his day and on the gross neglect exhibited by many of his fellow physicians. He also modestly admitted his own incompetence and, having declared that veterinary surgeons had more skill and were more successful in the treatment of old wounds than the most learned professors, went on to say, 'I wish I had their [the veterinary surgeons'] skill based on experience'.

An accolade indeed for our profession from the founder and master of the art of homoeopathy all those years ago. It has been a privilege to serve my chosen profession and I have been most fortunate to have enjoyed almost every minute of my life in general country practice. Homoeopathy has added another fascinating and most interesting chapter to my work.

SELECT BIBLIOGRAPHY

In writing this book the main sources consulted were:

Materia Medica with Repertory – W. Boericke, Boericke and Runyan, 1927.
Homoeopathic Drug Pictures – M. L. Tyler, Health Science Press, 1970.
Guide to Medicinal Plants – Schauenberg & Paris, Lutterworth Press, 1977.
Flora Homoeopathica – E. Hamilton, H. Bailliere, 1852 Reprinted by the Homoepathic Trust, 1981.
Keynotes and Characteristics with Comparisons – H. C. Allen, Thorsons Publishers, 1978.
Homoeopathic Green Medicine – A. C. Gordon Ross, Thorsons Publishers, 1978.
Homoeopathic Prescribing – N. Pratt, Beaconsfield Publishers, 1980.
Introduction to Homoeopathic Medicine – H. Boyd, Beaconsfield Publishers, 1981.

For those interested in the general subject of homoeopathy, the following two books are both 'good reads':

Homoeopathy by Dr G. Ruthven Mitchell, W. H. Allen, 1975.
The Patient, not the Cure by Dr M. Blackie, Macdonald, 1975.

INDEX